A-Z
NURSING

A-Z NURSING

Ms. Joshua Mathew

CENTRUM PRESS
NEW DELHI-110002 (INDIA)

CENTRUM PRESS
H.O.: 4360/4, Ansari Road, Daryaganj,
New Delhi-110 002 (India)
Ph.: 23278000, 23261597

B.O.: No. 1015, Ist Main Road, BSK IIIrd Stage
IIIrd Phase, IIIrd Block,
Bangalore - 560 085 (India)
Tel.: 080-41723429
Visit us at: www.centrumpress.com

A-Z Nursing

First Edition, 2009
ISBN 978-93-80106-03-8

PRINTED IN INDIA

Printed at Salasar Imaging Systems, Delhi-110035 (India)

Contents

Preface

Nursing theories are the creative products of nurses who seek to thoughtfully describe relationships and interactions that exist within nursing practice. The entire range of *private* nursing as distinguished from hospital nursing, and to instruct the nurse how best to meet the various emergencies of medical and surgical cases when distant from medical or surgical aid, or when thrown on her own resources, studiously refraining, however, from advising the nurse to act upon her own responsibility or to assume personal treatment of the patient except under circumstances of great urgency.

There is simply placed before the nurse what the different diseases are, their characters and chief points of distinction and the attention required, their possible complications, and the treatment likely to be adopted in a given case by the family physician, so that suitable preparations may be made by the nurse.

This method mobilizes creativity for the construction of personal meaning. In encouraging creativity through the use of the universal language of art, students become engaged and active learners. When this text and learning activities are used as a guide for learning, students do not sit passively in a classroom, memorizing definitions and facts. The activities outlined in this text are visual, tactile, and kinesthetic. Students are able to read, see, touch, and manipulate the learning materials. Although comprehensive understanding of theory is not the intent or result of this creative approach, a light of beginning understanding will be ignited by this approach.

Author

Chapter 1

Development of Nursing

ORIGIN AND GLOBAL PERCEPTION

The history of nursing spans from the history of human kind. For as long as there has been life, there has been the need to provide care and comfort to those suffering from illness and injury. From the dawn of civilization, evidence prevails to support the premise that nurturing has been essential to the preservation of life.

Survival of the human race, therefore, is in inextricably intertwined with the development of nursing. Nursing has been called the oldest of the arts and the youngest of the profession. The word nurse evolved from the Latin word nutritious, which means nourishing.

The roots of medicine and nursing are intertwining and found in mythology, ancient eastern and western cultures and religion. Nursing is defined by various authors at various times. Hansderson says "nursing is primarily assisting the individuals (sick or well) in the performances of those activities, contributing or its recovery (or to a peaceful death) that he would perform unaided, if he had the necessary strength, will or knowledge.

The unique contribution of nursing is to help the individual to be independent or such assistance as soon as possible. The International Council Of Nurses defines" Nursing is to assist the individual, sick or well in the performance of those activities contributing to health or to its recovery (or to peaceful death) that he would perform unaided if he had the necessary strength, will or knowledge. And to do this in such a way as to help in gain independence as rapidly as possible. Nursing, besides being a honourable profession, is one of the oldest arts and an essential modern occupation. Nursing is one of the greatest of humanitarian services and all people whether ill or well, rich or poor, literate or illiterate, young or old, at work or at play, in or out of hospital, are in some way or other, directly or indirectly closely associated with it. Nursing has its own body of knowledge scientifically based and humanitarianism that promises expanded benefits to people and society.

It assists the individual or family to achieve their potential for self-direction for health. Nursing is not only an applied science, it is also an art, which provides skillful care for the sick in appropriate relationship with the patient, family, physician and with others who have related responsibilities. It is concerned equally with the prevention of illness and the conservation of health.

Skillful nursing care embraces the whole person, body, mind and soul, his physical, mental, social and spiritual well-being (holistic approach). In its broadest sense, nursing covers not only the care of the sick, the aged, the helpless and the handicapped, but also cares for the promotion of health and prevention of illness.

The arts of nursing had its birth in the earliest home where a mother cared for the well being of the rest members of the family. It is this mother care that through the ages developed into a skilled art and a well-organized science. It will be interesting to know and understand the vast changes that nursing has passed through, in order to meet the needs of a changing civilization.

A study of the development of nursing will throw light on some of the problems of the past, how they have been solved and how nursing has progressed rapidly despite various hindrances. The paternal and maternal instinct in a human being is the main source of the nursing impulse, and is found in the hearts of people of all ages.

A mother's care for her sick child always found expression in such acts to alleviate pain and help the child to get better.

In a society, the noblest forms of humanitarianism are showing mercy, love and kindness to those in physical or mental distress. When this impulse or motive is re-enforced by religious philosophies and beliefs, it inspires people to live a life of service and of self-sacrifice for the sake of others. Along with this spirit, special training and experience has made nursing an ideal and useful profession.

PRE-HISTORIC NURSING

Myths, songs and other findings of the archaeologists throw some light on prehistoric man's care for this sick. In the pre-historic era, it was believed that illness was caused by evil spirits within the body. In order to get rid of the evil spirit, the body had to be illtreated. This was done by starving, beating, and administering nauseous medicines, beating of drums, magic rites and ceremonies and by causing sudden fright. Sometimes holes were made in the affected parts of the body to allow the evil spirit to escape.

Besides this, there were also many other ways of treating illness. Primitive man's skill in fighting disease has given us many medical and surgical treatments such as massage fomentations, trephining, bone setting, hot and cold baths, etc. The doctor cum nurse in such cases was the medicine man or the witch doctor or the priest physician.

NURSING IN EARLY CIVILIZATIONS

EGYPT

The Egyptians thought medicine to be of divine origin. One of the world's oldest medical records, dating back to 1600 B.C. comes from Egypt. Sources of medical history, description of diseases and their treatment, surgery and drugs used are found in the "Hieroglyphic writings" on papyrus from the temples of ancient Egypt and from the Pyramids.

Temple took the places of hospitals and the doctor cum nurse was the priest. It is probable that high-ranking women who become the priestesses in the temples played the role of nurses. Mothers and daughters nursed the sick at home. An outstanding priest physician was Imhotep. Because of his great love and kindness to his patients and of his success in healing, he was elevated to the rank of a deity. Embalming and bandaging of mummies led to the study of anatomy of the body and the study of various herbs and drugs in preservation of the same. The Egyptians recognised about 250 diseases and discovered suitable drugs and surgery for their treatment.

The sacred books were strictly followed by the priestphysicians. He was taken to task, if he deviated from the teaching of these books and if his patient dies. Even though Egypt had made much progress in medicine and nursing, it soon declined for no dissection was permitted and also no experiments in medicines were to be made. This together with the advent of the Romans led to its decline.

GREECE

Medicine was closely connected with religion in Greece as in India. According to Greek mythology, Apollo the Sun God was their God of healing. Asclepius, the son of Apollo, was the Greek God of medicine. The Greeks prayed to Apollo and Asclepius, and the goddess of health, Hygiea the daughter of Apollo for magical cures for their illnesses. Temples, where people came to worship were also places for the treatment of the sick and the priest-physician was in charge of them.

These temples were situated in a healthy location, in a cheerful and charming country-side with plenty of fresh air. In Greece, the emphasis was a positive health, in beauty and perfection - not sickness and misery.

The young of Athens were taught to give their bodies exquisite care. It was in Greece that personal hygiene developed to a degree never previously or subsequently approached. Much emphasis was given to personal cleanliness, exercise and dietetics rather than to matters of environmental sanitation. Hippocrates, 100 BC known as "Father of Scientific Medicine" had a medical foundation to start with. He found that health and prevention of disease depends on certain laws of nature. He also established an Ethical code of conduct for all who practiced medicine. Parts of his code are being used by medical students today and it forms the base of the `Nightingale's pledge'. He separated medicine from religion for the first time in the history. With the spreading of Greek 's influence in other countries, the Greeks introduced establishments that may be considered as modern city hospitals. They also established scientific methods of diagnosis and systematic methods of recording.

ROME

The Romans are best known for advances in public health. Rome had proper sanitation, drainage and sewage system, public baths and a type of public dispensary. The Roman noble women cared for the sick. With the advent of Christianity, deacons and deaconesses performed the duties of nurses. Galen, a Greek physician who lived in Rome about 100 BC, performed numerous experiments on animals to learn about anatomy and disease.

HEBREWS

The writings of Hebrews in the Old Testament speak about laws and principles of sanitation in accordance with modern bacteriology. They mention about selection of food, sanitation, segregation of the sick, disinfection and midwifery.

CHINA

The Chinese were well advanced in medicine and surgery. They had good knowledge of internal organs and knew about the circulation of the blood. They practiced dissection. They also practiced vaccination and physiotherapy. Liver for anaemia, seaweed for thyroid were administered. The sick were prayed for in halls of healing. Intestinal infection was prevented by drinking of tea. Much importance was given to cleanliness and hygiene.

INDIA

In India, we had the Ayurvedic system of medicine, which can be traced back to about 3000 B.C. Ayurveda stressed on hygiene, prevention of sickness, inoculation against small pox, sanitation, lavatories, good ventilation, kitchen, construction of hospitals, cultivation of medicinal plants and suitable building for housing animals. Atreya was the first great physician and teacher of Ayurveda.

He lived about 800 B.C. During 700-600 B.C Sushruta and Charaka started practice of surgery and medicine. Sushruta Samhita is written by the great surgeon Sushruta, who says "the physician, the patient, the drugs and the nurse are four feet of `Padas' of the medicine, upon which the cure depends". He then explains how cash may be a true `Pada' (Foot). The nurse is a pada when he is kindhearted, strong, trustworthy and mindful of the physician's orders.

The nurse is one who attends the patient; is cool headed and pleasant in his demeanour; does not speak ill of any body; is strong and attentive to the requirements of the sick and strictly follows the instructions of the physicians.

The great physician Charaka has written the Charaka Samhita in which he explains details of the manner in which drugs should be prepared or compounded for administration. According to him, resourcefulness, devotedness to the patient waited upon, and purity of mind and body are the qualification of the attending nurse.

The Charaka Samhita states that attendants on the sick should have good behaviour and should be distinguish for purity and cleanliness of habits. Nursing treatments prescribed are baths, enema to evacuate the bowels, emetics to produce vomiting, vaginal and urethral infusion (introducing a fluid under pressure), venesection (reducing of blood volume by opening the vein), gargles, massages, rubbing or pressing the limbs etc.

A nurse is expected to assist the patient to walk or move about. She/He must know how to make clean beds. She should be skilled in compounding drugs and ever willing to do any work that her profession demands of her. 700-600 B.C - Thiruvalluvar in his songs speaks highly of medicine. He describes medical care as consisting of patients, doctors and nurses. 264 B.C - King Ashoka made a great stride in the care of the sick, both human beings and animals. He not only founded a large number of hospitals for the sick but also made provision for the education and training of women for that purpose.

Monastery Universities were founded and became famous for their medical schools. The ethical standards of conduct demanded from those who attended upon the sick were of an exceptionally high order. The nursing of patients seems to have been devoted primarily to men, a great deal of unrewarded work. The qualities expected of nursing attendants were good behaviour, purity, cleverness, at kindness and skill.

EARLY CHRISTIAN ERA

Nursing in Pre-Christian times, religious beliefs had great bearing on the attitude towards the sick and the mode of caring for the sick and the suffering. Christianity believed that one should render services of love to humanity without any reward. It was equal to one's sincere love of God. This principle was absorbed in nursing and helped to improve the status of a nurse. Some of examples of such women are as follows:

Phoebe

She was the first deaconesses. She was intelligent and educated and the best nurse who could care fort the sick in their homes. She can be compared to a modern public health nurse.

Fabiola

She was a young, beautiful and attractive woman. She was the daughter of a great Roman Noble. She converted her palace into a hospital and it was the first Christian hospital in Rome. She collected the poor and sick from the streets and cared for them herself, in her place.

Paula

Paula was a friend of Fabiola. She devoted herself for the services of the sick. She built a hospital for strangers, pilgrims, and travellers and for the sick. She constructed a monastery in Bethlehem. They gave good nursing care for the sick.

Marcella

Marcella was a wealthy woman. Since women of high rank had much freedom in Rome, she was able to lead a group of such women and induce them in works of charity.

During the Middle Ages, monks and nuns devoted their life to the care and services of the poor and sick. The monasteries became the places of education, medical care and nursing. The following monks and the nuns devoted their life and services for the poor and the sick.

St. Dominic (1170-1221),

St. Francis of Assisi 1182 -1226.

St. Elizabeth of Hungary 1207 -1231

St. Catherine Sienna 1347 - 1380

The women who assisted in the work of clergy in the church were known as deaconesses. They were matured women, who did teaching, preaching and caring for the sick at the home. New thoughts and new ideas were introduced in the early Christian era.

Even though many religious were fatalistic in their out look on illness and looked upon it as a punishment or a necessary evil, Christianity introduced a new aspect on the subject, thus transforming nursing to a higher level and raising it to a professional standing.

This new aspect that of "altruism" was the highest motive given to mankind. It taught that one's sincere love for God and a desire to be like Him, would be the chief motive for one's selfless and sacrificial service to mankind without any hope of a reward. This inspired may godly men and women to step forward in the service of the sick, the suffering and the needy. They opened their homes to the sick and in need.

Such homes were called "Diakonia". During the time of the persecution of the Christians, people turned to the Bishop of the Church for help. This necessitated the building of homes cum hospitals where the strangers, the orphans, the aged, the sick and the lepers were cared for.

These homes cum hospitals were known as Xenodochia. One such outstanding hospital was founded at Casearia by St.Basil in 370 A.D. The Christian church preserved records and from that time till today we have a continuous record of the history of nursing. Many rich and noble women launched out in groups and organizations in the service of the sick and the ailing and used their wealth for this cause.

Monasteries came into being and became a heaven for those who needed help and care. Two notable names of people belonging to this era are worth mentioning. Celsius, a Greek, studied anatomy and knew how to do surgical operations for cataracts and hernias.

Galen practiced dissection on animals and studied the anatomy and physiology of the heart and circulation, the respiratory and the nervous system. His writings together with his translations of Hippocrates were considered to be the chief medical authority by the Arabs.

MIDDLE AGES

Monks and nuns dedicated to the cause of human suffering worked as doctors and nurses. They were skilled in the use of home remedies. They got scientific knowledge in the care of the sick from the books in the monasteries. They did the groundwork for the development of universities. In the later middle ages, many social problems presented themselves with the disintegration of the protective units like monasteries, guilds and feudalism and resulting in redistribution of population.

Late in the 12th and 13 th centuries nursing become differentiated from medicine and surgery. Medicine went into a period of advancement while nursing declined. At such time may noteworthy men and women came out to serve the sick. During the medieval period plague and pestilence were thought to be due to supernatural rather than natural causes. Religious expeditions like the crusades led to founding of secular as well as military hospitals.

Quarantine was instituted to check spreading of epidemics like plague. Social problems were solved to a great extent. The needs of abandoned children were met in hospital, leading to the founding of creches. People had an indifferent attitude towards sanitation and hygiene.

The Dark Ages was marked by superstition, mysticism, persecution of free thinkers and religious wares. Use of talisman and incantations for healing the sick become quite common.

THE DAWN OF MODERN NURSING

From the late 1700s through 1853, the manner in which the sick were cared, remain essentially unchanged. In Europe the dawn of nursing was underway. The Deaconess Institute of Kaiserswerth, Germany was established in 1836 by Pastor Theodor Fliedner, to train the Deaconesses to care for the sick and the provision of social services. Graduates of the Kaiserswerth programme spread their influence through out the world.

Florence Nightingale

Every one who had studied about Miss Florence Nightingale, knows of her devotion to the services to the poor and the sick and is also aware of what she did for humanity and to raise the status of nursing profession. Florence Nightingale was born in a wealthy English family, on 12th May 1820.

As she grew off, she became interested in people and in politics. She had great desire to become a nurse though her parents were not keen on her becoming one.

- She was dissatisfied with the dealt routine lifestyle of the upper class women of their days. She had an active mind and an interest in her surroundings beyond household and socials events.
- She had received a classical education equal to that of men of her day. This education provided her with an understanding of the circumstances of the world in which she lived.
- She became aware of the inadequate care being provided in hospitals, when she accompanied her mother on visits to the ill.

What Nightingale saw in the hospitals intrigued her and made her want to become more involved. In 1846, in spite of the concerns of parents and friends Nightingale became to visit and care for the sick in her community. In addition, she visited hospitals in England and throughout Europe. Out of her experiences she recognised that nurses required knowledge, training and discipline, if they were to be effective.

Nightingale learned about the school at Kaisersworth and in 1850, she was admitted to the training programme. The three years of training she received were rigorous but helped her clarify what was lacking in the current training of English nurses. After her training, in 1853 she was appointed as Superintendent of the Institution for the Care of the Sick Gentlewomen in London.

She had an opportunity to give her best service to the wounded soldiers in the Crimean War in 1854. Florence Nightingale and her nurses attended thousands of wounded and dying soldiers. Every night Florence Nightingale walked about with a lamp in her hand to help the suffering soldiers.

At this time she helped them to write letters to their families and last messages for those who were dying. She was rightly known as "The Lady with the Lamp". Nightingale and a small band of untrained nurses went to the British hospitals at Scutari in Turkey. She found the patients were laid on the floor in bloody uniforms.

Equipments and facilities were not present adequately. With great compassion, she set about the task of organizing and cleaning the hospital and provided care to the wounded soldiers. Through her efforts and the help of others, Nightingale introduced numerous improvements in the military hospital. Her efforts were largely responsible for traumatic reductions (42 per cent to 2per cent) in the wartime death rate of British Soldiers.

She also founded the first training school for nurses (St. Thomas Hospital, London, 1860). Throughout the publication of countless articles and papers, she shared her ideas about nursing and nursing education. Miss Nightingale was the first to mention Holism (treating the whole patient) in nursing and the first who stated that a unique body of knowledge is required to practice professional nursing.

After the war, she worked to bring about better health conditions in the British army. Nightingale almost single-handedly tried to change health care in England. Nightingale was the founder of modern nursing education. She established the Army Medical School at the Fort Pitt. Despite her ill health she worked for the development of nursing services without taking sufficient rest. Florence founded a training school for nurses in 1860 at St. Thomas Hospital London.

The funds, which were raised by the British people for her service in the Crimean War, were used for this training school. She was very much interested in improving the conditions of the army in India also.

She planned a complete public health programme, which was practiced in all hospitals and in the fields of nursing. She died peacefully in her sleep at the age of 90. In recognition of her meritorious help to mankind she was offered the Order of Merit in 1907.She was the first lady recipient for such an honour.

The Florence Nightingale Pledge

The modified Hippocratic Oath arranged by Mrs. Lystra E. Gretter and her committee for the Farrand Training School for Nurses, Detroit is called the Florence Nightingale Pledge as a token of esteem for the Founder of Modern Nursing. The pledge is taken by all the nurses who have completed the training programme before entering to their practice.

The Nurses Pledge

I solemnly pledge myself before God and in the presence of this assembly to pass my life in purity and to practice my profession faithfully. I will abstain from what ever is deleterious and mischievous and will not take or knowingly administer any harmful drug. I will do all in my power to maintain and elevate the standard of my profession and will hold the confidence in all personal matters committed to my keeping and all family affairs coming to my knowledge in the practice of my calling.

With loyalty, I will endeavor to aid the physician in his

work and devote myself to the welfare of those committed to my care.

The Renaissance or Revival of Learning in Europe

This was an age of discovery, invention, development, expansion and reorganization in all spheres of human life. It is said that in this period in Europe "The dignity of man began to be emphasized and the search for scientific truth was at least advocated." Curiosity about the natural world paved the way for rebirth of science.

There was great advancement in the science of health, science of chemistry, anatomy and great improvement in surgery. Many eminent people's discoveries and inventions led science to make great strides of progress in its various fields. Some of them were:

This age also emphasized on provision of pure water supply, proper disposal of refuse and adhering to sanitary laws. Boards of Health were set up for supervisory purposes.

NURSING IN INDIA

The ancient records of India indicate the principles and practices of nursing. They are so clear, intelligent and scientific, that many of them might fit into any of the modern textbook. The nurses were usually young men, and only in special cases, women were taken for conducting childbirth. The progress of nursing in India was obstructed by the low state of women, the caste system, illiteracy and political unrest. Military nursing was the earliest type of nursing. In 1664 the East India Company started a hospital for soldiers in a house at Fort St.George, Madras.

The first sisters were sent from St.Thomas Hospital, London to this military hospital. In 1797 a Lying - in - Hospital (maternity) for the poor of Madras was built with the help of subscriptions by Dr.John Underwood.

In 1854 the Government sanctioned a training school for midwives in Madras. Florence Nightingale was the first woman to have great influence over nursing in India and had a close knowledge of Indian conditions, especially army. She was interested in the nursing service for the civilian population, though her first interest was the welfare of the army in India.

In 1865, Miss Florence Nightingale drew up some detailed "Suggestions on a system of nursing for hospitals in India". Graduates were sent out from the Nightingale School of Nurses at St.Thomas Hospital, England to start similar schools in our country. St Stephens Hospital at Delhi was the first one to begin training the Indian girls as nurses in 1867. In 1871, the first School of Nursing was started in Government General Hospital, Madras with 6 months Diploma Midwives programme with four mid-wife students.

Four lady Superintendents and four trained nurses from England were posted to Madras. Between 1890 and 1900, many schools, under either missions or government, were started in various parts of India. In the yearly twentieth century, National Nursing Associations were started.

In 1897, Dr.B.C.Roy did great work in raising the standards of nursing and that of male and female nurses. In 1908, the trained nurses association of India was formed as it was felt to uphold the dignity and the honour of nursing profession.

In 1918, training schools were started for health visitors and dais, at Delhi and Karachi. Two English nurses Miss Griffin and Miss Graham were appointed to give training to and to supervise the nurses. In 1926, Madras State formed the first registration council to provide basic standards in education and training. The first four year basic Bachelor Degree programme were established in 1946 at the college of nursing in Delhi and Vellore.

With the assistance from the Rockfeller Foundations, seven health centers were set up between 1931 - 1939 in the cities of Delhi, Madras, Bangalore, Lucknow, Trivandrum, Pune and Calcutta. In 1947, after the independence, the community development programme and the expansion of hospital service created a large demand for nurses, auxiliary nurse midwives, health visitors, midwives, nursing tutors and nursing administrators.

The Indian Nursing Council was passed by our ordinance on December 31st 1947. The council was constituted in 1949. In 1956, Miss Adrenwala was appointed as the Nursing Advisor to Government of India. The development of Nursing in India was greatly influenced by the Christian missionaries, World War, British rule and by the International agencies such as W.H.O. Unicef, Red Cross, Unsaid etc.

The first master's degree course, a two-year postgraduate programme was begun in 1960 at the College of Nursing, Delhi. In 1963, the School of Nursing in Trivandrum, instituted the first two years post certificate Bachelor Degree programme. The associations such as International Council of Nurses, the nurses auxiliary of the CMA of India, T.N.A.I. Indian Nursing council and State level Registration Council are closely connected with promotion and the upliftment of the nursing profession.

Nursing in Tamilnadu

- In 1664 the East India Company started the first hospital at St. George, Madras.
- In 1797 a Lying-in-hospital for the poor of Madras was started.
- In 1854, the government sanctioned a Training School for running mid-wives course in Madras.

Training School

The first mid-wives School was started at the government hospital in 1871. The formal schools of nursing was started for conducting diploma in general nursing and mid-wifery programmes for a duration of 3 ½ years in Madras and in other parts of Tamilnadu. Schools of nursing offering diploma programme increased slowly (there were 9 schools of nursing and 4 mid-wifery schools till 2001) conducted by government of Tamilnadu.

The number of schools conducted by government of Tamilnadu is now increased to 17 in 2003 and now the government executed to start one school of nursing in every district hospitals. The numbers of private schools have also increased. Multipurpose health worker schools are also functioning in many places in Tamilnadu conducted by government and private bodies.

College of Nursing

A teachers training programme running for a duration of one year was functioning in government hospital. In 1967 an integrated 2-½ years Bachelor Science degree nursing programme attached to Madras Medical College (for trained nurses) commenced replacing the then existing diploma programme.

In 1980, diploma in community nursing programme was started. In 1983, Bachelor of Science Nursing, 4-year programme was started in College of Nursing, attached to Madras Medical College. In 1995, Master of Science (Nursing) programme was started in the College of Nursing, attached to Madras Medical College.

In 2001, a post of Principal for the College of Nursing was sanctioned and started functioning. Dr. Sumathi Kumarswamy was appointed as the first Principal. Many candidates have completed Doctoral degree in nursing. In 2003, a College of Nursing at Madurai started functioning by the government.

Services

The cadre strength of nursing increased slowly and many categories in nursing services prompted up. In 1962, a post of Assistant to Director of Medical Services was created and filled at the state level. A post of Deputy Director of Nursing at the state level was created in 1986, and Dr Sumathi Kumaraswamy was appointed as the first Deputy Director of Medical Education in Nursing in 1992.

The Development of Auxiliary Nurse Midwife Training (Rural Health Services)

During the Second World War, there was a great demand for nursing personnel in the military hospitals as well as in the civil hospitals. So auxiliary nurses midwife services was founded in 1942. This course was simple and the duration of training period was shorter than the nursing course. The nurses under this course were posted to do useful work under supervision in the hospital, or in the health centre and to give domiciliary care.

Auxiliary nurse midwives were prepared to meet the demands of the health personnel in the community development programmes. After the independence and in the Second Five Year Plan, it was decided to prepare six thousand auxiliary nurses and midwives. The private hospitals also were requested to co-operate with the Government to start such training institution. The government hospitals were given facilities to train the auxiliary nurse midwife since 1955.

Today the auxiliary nurse midwife has a vital role in the health services of the rural health centers such as primary health centre, family welfare centre, Maternity and Child Health centers. They can work as a midwife and a health worker in the community. They are also given opportunity to be trained as health visitors or as nurses if they have the basic educational requirements.

The practice of the auxiliary nurse midwife in the rural centre had helped to improve the health status of the people, by health teaching, domiciliary care, and regular follow-up of patients and families. Auxiliary nurse midwife in the present health care delivery system functions as a Multipurpose Female Health Worker.

With the present introduction of vocational courses such as nursing in the academic stream as one of the options, it is believed that it will contribute towards the basic nursing care of individuals, families and community for health and happiness. It will also be a foundation course for future diploma and degree programs in nursing.

SCOPE OF NURSING

There was a time when professional nurses had very little choice of service because nursing was centered in the hospital and bedside nursing. Career opportunities are more varied now for a numbers of reasons. The list of opportunities available are given under:

- Staff Nurse provides direct patient care to one patient or a group of patients. Assists ward management and supervision. She is directly responsible to the ward supervisor.
- Ward sister or Nursing Supervisor, She is responsible to the nursing superintendent for the nursing care management of a ward or unit. Takes full charge of the ward.

  Assigns work to nursing and non-nursing personnel working in the ward. Responsible for safety and comfort of patients in the ward. Provides teaching sessions if it is a teaching hospital.
- Department supervisor/Assistant Nursing Superintendent. She is responsible to the nursing superintendent and deputy nursing superintendent for the nursing care and management of more than one ward or unit. Example-Surgical department. Out-patient department.
- Deputy nursing superintendent. She is responsible to the nursing superintendent and assists in the nursing administration of the hospital.
- Nursing Superintendent She is responsible to the medical superintendent for safe and efficient management of hospital nursing services.
- Director of Nursing She is responsible for both nursing service and nursing educations within a teaching hospital.
- Community Health Nurse (CHN) services rendered mainly focusing Reproductive Child Health programme.
- Teaching in nursing. The functions and responsibilities of the teacher in nursing are planning, teaching and supervising the learning experiences for the students. Positions in nursing education are clinical instructor, tutor, senior tutor, lecturer, and associate professor, Reader in nursing and Professor in nursing.
- Industrial nurse Industrial nurses are providing first

aid, care during illness, health educations about industrial hazards and prevention of accidents.

- Military Nurse. Military Nursing service became a part of the Indian Army by which means nurses became commissioned officers who are given rank from liutenant to major general.
- Nursing service abroad Attractive salaries and promising professional opportunities, which causes a major increase for nursing service in abroad.
- Nursing service administrative positions. At the state level the Deputy Director of Nursing at the state health directorate. The highest administrative position on a national level is the Nursing Advisor to the Govt. of India.

Nursing in India - A Global Perception: If we are aware of current trends it will help us plan for developments in nursing education and nursing services as well as controlling the direction in which the profession moves. A global perception will enable nurses to rise to higher levels in their knowledge, skills and improved performance both in India and around the globe.

The Factors Influencing the Trends in Nursing

Changes in Society

For the past five decades, five social factors have greatly influenced present trends in nursing. These are,

- Intensive efforts of government to meet the health needs of people.
- Gradual improved literacy level of the people with the growing awareness of health needs.
- Advanced scientific technology
- The changing role of women and
- The continuing growth of population.

Changes in other professions.

Trends in the nursing profession have always been closely related to those in the medical profession. Growing specialization in medical field is resulting in a trend towards increased specialization in nursing. The development of new diagnostic procedure and equipments make specialization even more necessary.

Patients Bill of Rights

After the development of the "Patients Bill of Rights", the nurses are also accountable for patients care and have legal responsibilities for the patient.

Developments in other Discipline

Developments in other discipline other than medicine also influence trends in nursing profession.

Nursing is moving towards more specific nursing functions as other members of health team like dieticians, social workers and physiotherapists are more available and more highly specialized.

Leadership Within the Profession

Leadership within the profession also influences the trends in nursing. Nursing is moving towards professionalism due to the untiring efforts of nurses who have been dedicated to achieve the aim.

Working and Studying in Abroad

Working and studying in abroad is influenced by many factors within India and in other countries. Shortage of nurses in other countries, higher salary paid in abroad is the main causes for the working of Indian nurses in abroad.

Greater Specialization in Nursing Education and Practice

Greater specialization in nursing education and practice is a trend related to that in the medical profession and the growing amount of scientific knowledge available.

Working Conditions

Working conditions for nurses are also changing. There is a gradual change towards shorter and more convenient hours of duty, better accommodations and higher salaries.

Trends in other Countries

Trends in other country also influence the trends in the nursing profession in India. The rapid development of the degree programme has promoted the same emphasis and development here for professional nursing.

Changing roles and Functions of the Nurse as Perceived in the Globe

The nurses in India are also prepared and more privileged to face the changes and ready to accept the challenging roles and functions of the nurse as perceived in the globe because of the development in the education and training system. The following roles and positions perceived as in the globe are given below.

- Nurse educator works in schools of nursing, staff development departments. They provide the educational programme for student's nurses and nurses, teach clients about the self-care and home care.
- Clinical nurse specialist specializes in managing specific diseases and they function as clinicians, educators, managers, consultants and researchers.
- Nurse practitioners are certified to provide health care to clients in out-patient or community settings.
- Certified nurse-midwife are certified by the American College of Nurse-Midwives to provide independent care for women during normal pregnancy, labour and delivery.
- Nurse anesthetist, having advance training in anesthesiology, provides surgical anesthesia to the client under the supervision of an anesthesiologist during minor surgery with baccalaureate degrees or master's degree.
- Nurse administrators manage client care within the healthcare agencies in a middle level or upper level management position.
- Nurse researcher with Doctoral degree investigate nursing problem to improve care and to define and

expand the scope of nursing practice. Advancements in science increase health needs of the society and thereby expect changes in the role of nurses and thus increases the scope for nurses.

Ethics in Nursing

The Oxford dictionary defines ethics as "a science of human duty in its widest extent." The Chambers describes it as "the science of morals, that branch of philosophy which is concerned with human character and conduct." Webster defines it as "the morals concerned with or relating to what is right and wrong in matters of human behaviour." A code is needed to educate and orient members of the profession to distinguish desirable from the undesirable behaviours, to regulate relationships with co-workers and clients, and to guide the public in understanding professional conduct."

A group of nurses stated, "Ethics is knowledge and attitudes that determine man's relationship to himself, to others and to the society." Ethics is a science that endeavors to interpret the highest standards of written or unwritten principles or doctrines or morals of human duty, human character and conduct of human behaviour and human relationships in day-to-day life.

Ethics in nursing is a particular code of behaviours, characters, conducts and relationship unique only to the nursing personnel. Nursing ethics is "a system of principles governing the conduct of a nurse, her relationship to the patient and his family, her associates and society at large." As a guidelines to all those in the nursing profession, the Grand Council of the International Council of Nurses held at Sao Paulo, Brazil on July 10, 1953, adopted, viewed and revised in the year 1964.

Code of Ethics as Applied to Nursing

The codes of ethics are as follows:

- The nurse provides services with respect for human dignity irrespective of social or economic status, personal attributes, or the nature of health problems

- The fundamental responsibility of the nurse is threefold; to conserve life, to alleviate suffering and to promote health.
- The nurse shall maintain at all time the highest standards of nursing care and of professional conduct.
- The nurse must not only be well prepared to practice but shall maintain knowledge and skills at a consistently high level.
- The religious beliefs of a patient shall be respected.
- Nurses hold in confidence all personal information entrusted to them.
- Nurses recognise not only the responsibilities but the limitations of their professional functions not to recommend or give medical treatment without medical orders except in emergencies, and report such action to a physician as soon as possible.
- The nurse is under an obligation to carry out the physician's orders intelligently and loyally and to refuse to participate in unethical procedures.
- The nurse assumes responsibility and accountability for individual nursing judgments and actions.
- The nurse sustains confidence in the physician and other members of the health team; incompetence or unethical conduct of associates should be exposed but a only to the proper authority.
- The nurse safeguards the patients and the public when health care and safety are affected by the incompetent, unethical or illegal practice of any person.
- The nurse co-operates with the health team and maintains harmonious relationships with members of other professions and with nursing colleagues.
- The nurse adheres to standards of personal ethics, which reflect credit upon the profession.
- In personal conduct nurses should not knowingly disregard the accepted pattern of behaviours of the community in which they live and work.

- The nurse participates and shares responsibility with other citizens and other health professions in promoting forts to meet the health needs of the public - local, state, national and international.

Requests poured in from many quarters of the nursing world to review and revise this code against and representation for this purpose was made thorough several national councils.

In accordance with these requests the Professional Service Committee of the ICN selected a sub-committee for the revision of the code. The final revised code was submitted to the ICN Council of National Representatives in Mexico in May 1973 at the 15th Quadrennial congress. The Sub-committee on the Code of Ethics tried to concentrate their attention on the most vital aspects of nursing and built their revised ethical code around five major headings.

- *Nurses and people:* Nurse's responsibility is to those people who require nursing care. A person's values, customs and religious beliefs must be respected. Personal information must be held in confidence or shared only with judgments.
- *Nurses and Practice:* The nurse is responsible for giving the best care possible at all times and under all circumstances and maintaining a high standard of practice.
- *Nurses and Society:* The Code states the responsibility of the nurse for positive promotion health of the society by initiating and supporting action to meet the health and social needs
- *Nurses and co-workers:* The nurse is the member of the health team which is made up of all those who serve to meet the health needs of people. Nurses are expected to cooperate and to work well with nursing colleagues, the other members of the health team and members of other health professions.
- *Nurses and the profession:* The Code points out very clearly the role of the nurse as a leader and an active participator in professional activities by setting up

and carrying out desirable standards of nursing practice and nursing education.

Qualities of a Professional Nurse

For an efficient discharging of her/his duties and for a satisfactory fulfillment of all the aims and aspirations that her/his profession stands for, the following qualities in a nurse are inevitable.

- *Love:* with all its other attendant qualities like mercy, kindness, gentleness, patience and understanding are a must in a successful nurse. All her service for the sick and disabled are sponsored by these qualities. Without these essential characteristics the nurse becomes only a mechanical aid.
- *Willingness and self-sacrifice:* These two qualities are complimentary to each another. Because she is willing to serve under any trying situation, a nurse sacrifices her time, comfort and even material benefits. Eg. Florence Nightingale at Scutari.
- *Reliability:* A nurse is one who can be depended upon for a faithful discharging of her duties, the patients under her care, their families, doctors and members of the "health team" depend on her, for she is trust worthy and competent.
- *Resourcefulness:* In critical circumstances she uses her wisdom and knowledge and performs her duties to the best of her ability with whatever means that are at her disposal. She tackles situations with alacrity.
- *Courage:* In times of confusion, calamity or catastrophe, the nurse manages her work with compassion and is ready to meet any problem with courage. She is cool and levelheaded and does not get agitated easily.
- *Loyalty and honesty:* Her relationship with the patient, the doctor and her associates are marked by utmost loyalty and honesty.
- *Observant:* A good nurse is always vigilant. She keeps a close and constant watch on the patients, their

progress, their changes and reactions to treatment etc. and gives the doctor timely reports, A nurse should anticipate and meet the patients' needs.

- *Willingness to learn:* A nurse must keep in touch with the latest discoveries and developments in medicine and treatment and must "maintain her knowledge and skill at a consistently high level".
- *Co-operative and considerate:* A nurse learns to live in harmony with patients, doctors and other members of the health team and tries to help them in times of need.
- *Cleanliness:* A nurse is always clean and neat personally and in her work. She must be tidy and demand high standards of cleanliness from those whom she is associated within her profession.
- *Spirituality:* A nurse must learn to create a spiritual atmosphere for the patient and must try and help the patients to put their confidence and trust in a "Power" that is higher than any other power in the world.

Nursing as a Profession - A New Perspective. Historically, only medicine, law and the ministry were accepted as profession.

Criteria of a Profession

Genevieve and Roy Bixler first wrote about the status of nursing as a profession in 1945. These criteria include the following.

- The services provided are vital to humanity and the welfare of the society. Nursing is the service that is essential to the wellbeing of the people and to the society. Nursing promotes, maintains and restores the health of individuals, groups and communities. Assisting others to attain the highest level of wellness is the goal of nursing. Caring, meaning nurturing and helping others are the basic components of professional nursing.
- There is a special body of knowledge that is

continually enlarged through research. In the past, nursing was based on principles borrowed from the physical and social sciences and other disciplines. Today there is a unique body of knowledge to nursing.

- The services involve intellectual activities. Individual responsibilities (accountability) are a strong feature. Nursing has developed and refined its own unique approach to practice. Nursing process is a cognitive activity that requires both critical and creative thinking and serves as the basis of providing nursing care. Individual accountability in nursing has become the hallmark of practice.

  Accountability is ' is being answerable to some one for something one has done' Through legal opinion and court cases, society has demonstrated that nurses are individually responsible for their actions as well as for those of personnel under their supervision.
- Practitioners are educated in institution of higher learning. There are basic nursing programme, baccalaureate programme, masters and Doctoral programme in nursing
- Practitioners are relatively independent and control their own policies and activities. (Autonomy). Autonomy or control over one's practice is another controversial area for nursing. Although many nursing actions are independent, most nurses are employed in hospitals where authority resides in one's position.
- Practitioners are motivated by service (altruism) and considered their work an important component of their lives. Nurses are dedicated to the ideal of service to others, which is known as altruism
- There is a Code of Ethics to guide the decisions and conduct of practitioners. The International Council of Nurses (ICN) has established Code of Nursing Ethics through which standards of practice are established, promoted and refined.

- There is an organisation (Association) that encourages and supports high standards of practice. Nursing has a number of professional associations that were formed to promote the improvement of the profession. Foremost among these, is the TNAI (The Trained Nurses Association of India). The purposes of TNAI are to foster high standards of nursing practice, promote professional and educational advancement of nurses and promote the welfare of the nurses.

Professional Organisations

Organisations provide a means through which united efforts are made to elevate standards of nursing education and practice. It also offers a means of voicing and opinions, developing our abilities and keeping informed of new trends.

The Indian Nursing Council (INC)

The Indian Nursing Council was authorized by the Indian Nursing Council Act of 1947. It was established in 1949 to provide uniform standards in nursing education and reciprocity in nursing registration throughout the country.

Functions

- It provides uniform standards in nursing education and reciprocity in nursing registration.
- It has authority to prescribe curriculum for nursing education in all states.
- It has authority to recogonise programme of nursing education or to refuse recognition of a programme if it did not meet the standards required by the council.
- It is registering the foreign nurses.
- It also maintains the Indian Nurses Register.
- The INC authorises State Nurses Registration Council and examining boards to issue qualifying certificates.

The International Council of Nurses (ICN)

The International Council of Nurses was founded in 1899

by Mrs. Bedford Fenwick.It is federation of non-political and self-governing national nurses association. The ICN is the global voice of nursing. The main purpose of the ICN is to provide the means through which the national associations can share their interests in the promotion of health and care of the sick.

Objectives of ICN

- To promote the development of the strong national nurses association.
- To assist national nurses association to improve the standards of nursing education and practice.
- To assist national nurses association to improve the status of nurses within their countries.
- To serve as the authoritative voice for nurses and nursing internationally.

Activities

- The ICN has published the Code for Nurses
- It makes the policy statement on health and social issues.
- It also maintains and improves the status of nurses and standard of nursing around the world.
- The council works to improve the nursing education and practice by publishing the guidelines for National Nurses Association.

The governing body of the ICN is the Council of National Representatives, which is made up of the ICN honorary officers and the presidents of the national member associations. The ICN publishes the International Nursing Review and the News Letter, which give the news of the ICN and the National Member Association.

TamilNadu Nurses and Mid-wives Council: Every professional nurses in the nursing professions, either here or abroad must be registered with the one of the State Nurses Registration Councils. The state council functions as an official to control the standards of the nursing practice

Activities

- It registers Nurses/Mid-wives
- It serves as legal protections to the nurses

- It protects the public from incompetent nursing practices or poor nursing care.
- It accredits and inspects schools of nursing and college of nursing.
- It prescribes the rules of conduct, take disciplinary action etc.
- It takes united efforts to elevate the standards of nursing.
- It works for the welfare of the members.

*World Health Organization (Who):*The World Health Organization is a specialized agency of the United Nations. It was organized in 1948 to achieve the highest possible level of health for all people. More than 150 countries are members of Who and help to finance the financial requirement the health care activities around the world. The Who is also active in nursing education and practice in a number of ways in India:

- It has offered guidance in setting up programme of nursing education
- It has promoted training for auxiliary nursing personnel
- The Who promotes public health in many ways around the world

The International Red Cross Society: The International League of Red Cross was formed in 1919 after World War I. It was closely with national societies during times of national disasters, providing expertise and conducting seminars to help these societies to improve their administrations and services.

A super global body made up of the above League and national societies is the International Conference of Red Cross's activities. The body meets once in four years. It supports unity in the work of all of these originations and promotes governmental support of the Red Cross Activities

The Indian Red Cross Society: The Indian Red Cross Society was established in 1920, with major aims of helping others from a neutral point. It gives relief to needy and suffering people at times of major disasters and in times of wars.

Aims: Prevention of disease, promotion of health and care of the sick in any kind of situation.

Functions

- Gives financial aid to social welfare institutions
- Operates blood banks through out India
- It teaches first aid

United Nations International Children's Educational Fund (Unicef): unicef is an agency of the United Nations. It was founded in 1946 for the purpose of helping mothers and children in country affected by World War II. Now it offers services in all underdeveloped countries. Unicef in India has provided teaching equipments for nursing education, textbooks and visual aids for schools and colleges of nursing and training for personal to help .with the health of mothers and children. *Trained Nurses Association in India (TNAI):* The trained Nurses Association of India is a largest national professional association of nurses in India.It was established in 1922. Aims of Trained Nurses Association in India (TNAI)

- Upholding the dignity and honour of the nursing profession.
- Promoting the sense of unity among all nurses
- Enabling members to discuss together on matters relating to their profession

*Student Nurses Association of India (SNA):*The student Nurses Association organised in 1929 is associated under the jurisdiction of the TNAI, in addition to providing a means of personnel and professional development for the nursing students. It serves as a source of membership for the parent organisation. In addition the TNAI serves as the advisor for the SNA.

Functions of SNA

The functions of SNA are as follows:

- To help the student nurses learn how the professional organisations serve to uphold the dignity and the ideals of the nursing profession.
- To furnish student nurses, in the courses of study leading to professional qualification.

*Christian Medical Association of India:*The Nurse's League of the Christian Medical Association was founded in 1930.

The current objectives:

- To promote co-operation and encouragement among Christian nurses.
- To promote efficiency in nursing education and services.
- To secure the highest standard possible in Christian Nursing Education through the Christian Schools of Nursing and
- To consider the special work and problems of Christian nurses working. Nursing considered to be an occupation now attains the status of profession.

NURSING AND HEALTH CARE DELIVERY SYSTEM IN INDIA

Nursing is a major component of the health care delivery system and nurses make up the largest employment group within the system. Nursing services are necessary for every patient seeking care of various types including primary, secondary, tertiary and restorative.

As nursing is an important part of health care delivery system, the nurses need to understand the system to effectively deliver quality care within it. Nursing is the process of recognizing, understanding and meeting the health needs of any person or society and is based on a constantly changing body of scientific knowledge.

*Nursing Process:*It is a deliberate intellectual activity whereby the practice of nursing is approached in an orderly, systematic manner to patient care, in a dynamic, continuous method to assist the patient to achieve and maintain health. T he nursing process is an orderly systematic manner of determining the patient' s problems, making plans to solve them, initiating the plan or assigning others to implement it and evaluating the extent to which the plan was effective in resolving the problems identified.

The nursing process is a systematic method for assessing health status, diagnosing health care needs, formulating a plan of care, initiating plan and evaluating the effectiveness of plan. The nursing process consists of five interrelated phases

- Assessment
- Diagnosis
- Planning
- Implementation
- Evaluation

Assessment: This refers to a systematic collection of data, to assist in identifying needs and problems. Data are collected in a systematic fashion, utilizing the interview or nursing history, physical examinations, laboratory results and other resources.

Diagnosis: Nursing diagnosis is a clinical judgment about individual family or community responses to actual and potential health problems and life processes. During this phase, the data collected during assessment are critically analysed and interpreted. Conclusions are drawn regarding the patient's needs, problems, concerns and human responses.

Planning: Planning is a systematic approach in developing a plan of action based on a careful assessment. Strategies are developed to prevent, minimize or connect the problems identified in the nursing diagnosis. It consists of several steps including establishing priorities, setting objectives, writing interventions, recording outcomes of nursing interventions in an organized fashion to complete the nursing care plan.

Implementation: It refers to carry out a plan that is based on careful assessment of need. It is the initiation and completion of action necessary to achieve the outcomes or objectives.

Evaluation: It is an ongoing process that determines the extent to which the goals care has been achieved. The nurses assess the progress of the patient, institute corrective measures if required, and revise the nursing care plan.

ADVANTAGES OF NURSING PROCESS

The nursing process helps the nurse and the nursing in many ways

- Helps to create a health data base of a patient
- Helps to identify actual or potential health problems of a patient

- Helps to establish priorities of nursing actions for providing proper services to the patients.
- Helps to define specific nursing actions for providing proper services to the patients
- Helps to develop planned organized and individualised nursing care.
- Helps to encourage for innovative nursing care.
- Helps to provide for alternative nursing actions.
- Helps to develop nursing autonomy and to foster nursing accountability
- Helps to increase the effectiveness of nursing care.

Health: World Health Organization (Who) defines health as a " state of completes physical, mental and social wellbeing, not merely the absence of disease or infirmity.

Illness: I t is a state in which a person' s physical, emotional, intellectual, social or spiritual functioning is diminished or impaired.

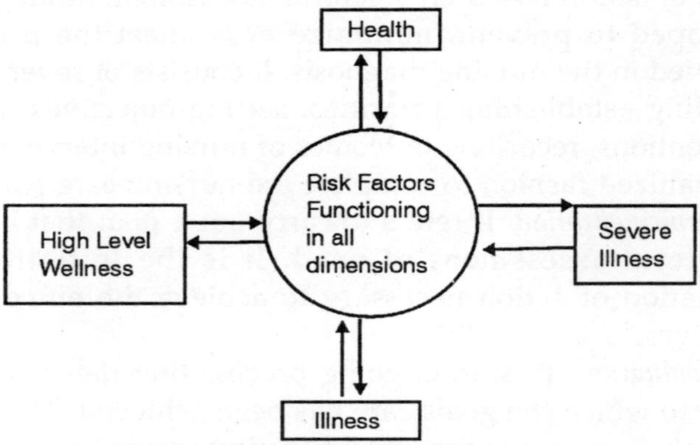

Fig. Health - Illness Continuum

Health - illness continuum: Health is a dynamic state that fluctuates as a person adapts to changes in the internal and external environments to maintain a state of wellbeing.

As health and illness are relative qualities existing in varying degrees, it is more accurate to consider health and illness in terms of a scale or continuum, rather than a absolute state.

VARIABLES INFLUENCING HEALTH BELIEFS AND PRACTICES

Internal Variables

- *Developmental stage:* A person ' s thought and behaviour patterns change throughout life.
- *Intellectual background:* Knowledge about body functions and illnesses, educational background and past experiences, all influence the health beliefs and practice of patients.
- *Emotional and spiritual factors:* The patient ' s degree of calm or stress can influence health beliefs and practices. Spiritual beliefs also influence whether and how a patient seeks or avoids healthy behaviour.

External Variables

- *Family Practices*: The way that patient' s families use health care services, their perceptions of the seriousness of diseases and their preventative care behaviours can influence the health beliefs and practice.
- *Socioeconomic Factors*: Social relationships, economic level and psychosocial factors influence health beliefs and practice.
- *Cultural background*: It influences beliefs, values and customs. It influences the approach to the health care system, personal health practices and nurse-patient relationship.

FACTORS AFFECTING A PATIENT' S HEALTH STATUS

- Smoking
- Nutrition
- Alcohol use
- Habituating drug use
- Driving
- Exercise
- Sexuality and contraceptive use

- Family relationships
- Risk factor modification
- Coping and adaptation.

IMPACT OF ILLNESS ON PATIENT AND FAMILY

Impact of Illness on Patient

Short - term and minor illnesses awoke few behavioural changes in the functioning of the patient or family. Severe illness can lead to more extensive emotional and behavioral changes such as anxiety, shock, denial, anger and withdrawal.

Impact on Family Roles

When an illness occurs, the role of patients and family may change. This change may be subtle and short term or drastic and long term.

The patient and family require specific counseling and guidance to assist them in coping with the role changes during illness.

HEALTH CARE DELIVERY SYSTEM IN INDIA

In dia is a union of 28 states and 7 union territories. States are largely independent in matters relating to the delivery of health care to the people. Each state has developed its own system of health care delivery, independent of the Central Government.

The Central Government responsibility consists mainly of policy making, planning, guiding, assisting, evaluating and coordinating the work of the State Health Ministries. The health system in India has 3 main links

- Central
- State and
- Local or peripheral

At the centre: T h e official "organs" of the health system at the national level consist of

- Ministry of Health and Family Welfare
- The Directorate General of Health Services
- The Central Council of Health and Family Welfare

Union Ministry of Health and Family Welfare

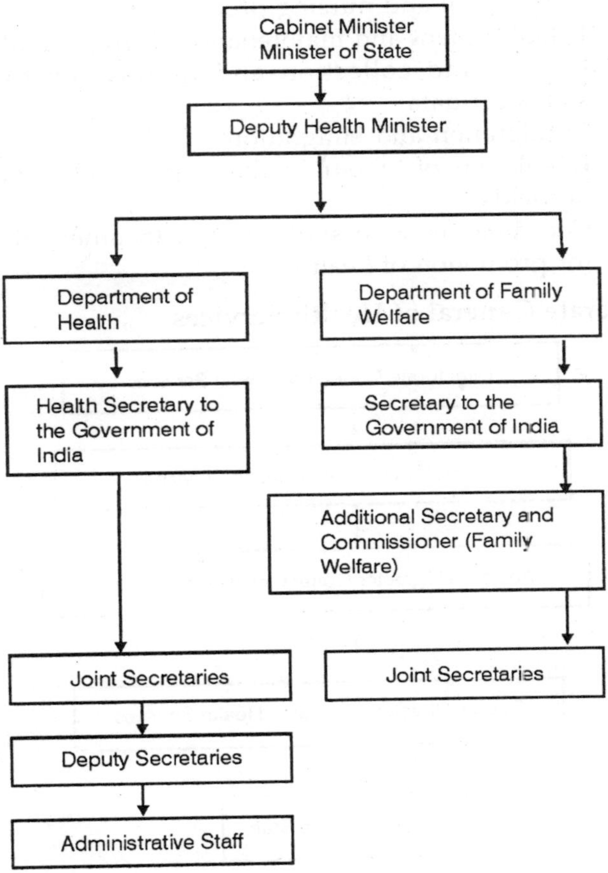

Fig. Organization Pattern

Functions

Union list

- International health relations and administration of port quarantine
- Dminisration of Central Institutes such as All India Institute of Hygiene and Public Health, Kolkata.
- Promotion of research through research centers

- Regulation and development of medical, pharmaceutical, dental and nursing professions
- Establishment and maintenance of drug standards
- Census and collection and publication of other statistical data
- Immigration and emigration
- Regulation of labour in the working of mines and oil fields
- Coordination with states and with other ministries for promotion of health

Directorate General of Health Services

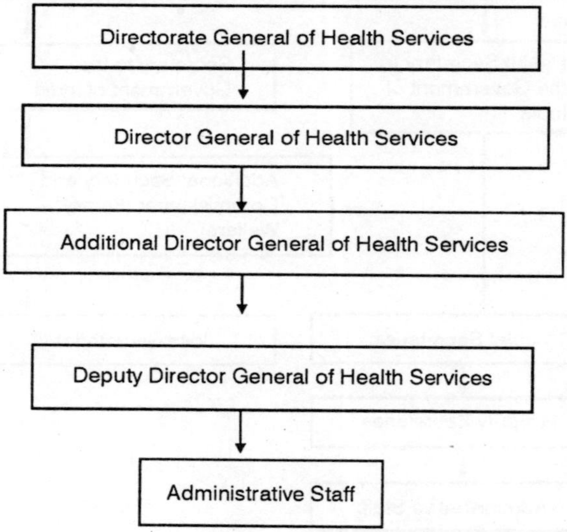

Fig. Organization Pattern

Concurrent list

The functions listed under the concurrent list are the responsibility of both the union and state governments

- Prevention and extension of communicable diseases
- Prevention of adulteration of food stuffs
- Control of drugs and poisons
- Vital statistics
- Labour welfare

- Ports other than major
- Economic and social planning
- Population control and Family Planning

Functions

- International health relations and quarantine of all major ports in country and international airport
- Control of drug standards
- Maintain medical store depots
- Administration of post graduate training programmes
- Administration of certain medical colleges in India
- Conducting medical research through Indian Council of Medical Research (ICMR)
- Central Government Health Schemes.
- Implementation of national health programmes
- Preparation of health education material for creating health awareness through Central Health Education Bureau.
- Collection, compilation, analysis, evaluation and dissemination of information through the Central Bureau of Health Intelligence
- National Medical Library

Central Council of Health

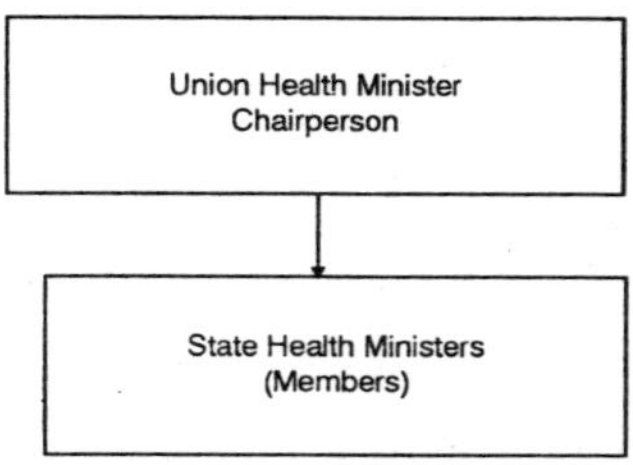

Fig. Organisation Pattern

Functions

- To consider and recommend broad outlines of policy regard to matters concerning health like environment hygiene, nutrition and health education.

- To make proposals for legislation relating to medical and public health matters.
- To make recommendations to the Central Government regarding distribution of grants-in-aid.

At the State Level

The health subjects are divided into three groups: federal, concurrent and state. The state list is the responsibility of the state, including provision of medical care, preventive health services and pilgrimage within the state.

STATE HEALTH ADMINISTRATION

At present there are 28 states in India, each state having its own health administration

State Ministry of Health

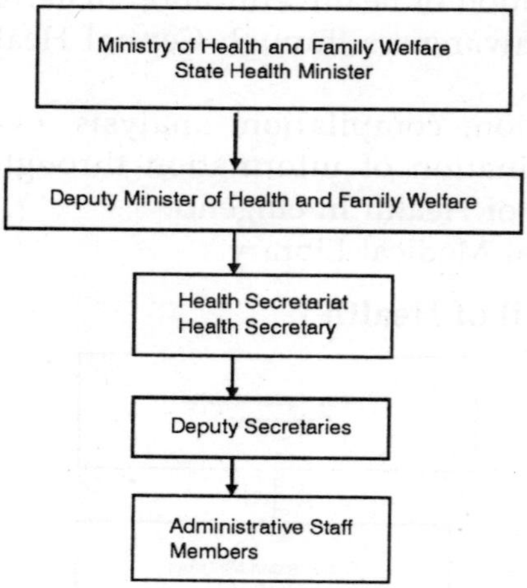

Fig. Organization Pattern

State Health Directorate

Two separate major departments, medical and public health are functioning in the state

- The Directorate of Health Services or the Director of Medical and Health Services

- The Directorate of Health and Family Welfare
- The Directorate of Medical Education for the management of medical colleges and hospitals.
- The Directorate of Public Health Services

AT THE DISTRICT LEVEL

There are 593 (year 2001) districts in India. Within each district, there are 6 types of administrative areas.

- Sub-division
- Tehsils (Taluks)
- Community Development Blocks
- Municipalities and Corporations
- Villages and
- Panchayats
  - Most district in India are divided into two or more subdivision, each incharge of an Assistant Collector or Sub Collector
  - Each division is again divided into taluks, incharge of a Thasildhar. A taluk usually comprises between 200 to 600 villages
  - The community development block comprises approximately 100 villages and about 80000 to 1,20,000 population, in charge of a Block Development Officer.
  - Finally, there are the village panchayats, which are institutions of rural local self-government.
  - The urban areas of the district are organized into
  - Town Area Committees (in areas with population ranging between 5,000 to 10,000)
  - Municipal Boards (in areas with population ranging between 10,000 and 2,00,000)
  - Corporations (with population above 2,00,000)
  - The Town Area Committees are like panchayats. They provide sanitary services.
  - The Municipal Boards are headed by Chairmen/ President, elected by members.

The Functions of Municipal Board

- Construction and maintenance of roads

- Sanitation and drainage
- Street lighting
- Water supply
- Maintenance of hospitals and dispensaries
- Education and
- Registration of births and deaths etc
- The Corporations are headed by Mayors, elected by councillors, who are elected from different wards of the city.

The executive agency includes the commissioner, the secretary, the engineer and the health officer. The activities are similar to those of municipalities, on a much wider scale.

Panchayat Raj

The panchayat raj is a 3-tier structure of rural local self-government in India, linking the village to the district

- Panchayat (at the village level)
- Panchayat Samiti(at the block level)
- Zila Parishad(at the district level)

Panchayat (at the Village Level)

- The Panchayat Raj at the village level consists of
- The Gram Sabha
- The Gram Panchayat
- The Gram Sabha considers proposals for taxation, and elects members of The Gram Panchayat.
- The Gram Panchayat covers the civic administration including sanitation and public health and work for the social and economic development of the village.

Panchayat Samiti (at the Block Level)

- The Panchayat Samiti execute the community development programme in the block. The Block Development Officer and his staff give technical assistance and guidance in development work.

Zila Parishad (at the District Level)

- The Zila Parishad is the agency of rural local

selfgovernment at the district level. Its functions and powers vary from state to state.

Types of Health Care Agencies

Health care is provided in various settings.

- *Out Patient Services*: Patients who don require hospitalization can receive health care in a clinic. An out patient setting is designed to be convenient and easily accessible to the patient. Hospital Settings (To get the material) Out patient services are generally directed at primary and secondary health centers.
- *Clinics*: Clinics involve a department in a hospital where patients not requiring hospitalization, receive medical care.
- *Institutions:* Hospitals-Hospital have been the major agency of health care system. Hospitals are classified as
  - Public
  - Private
  - Military

A Public Hospital are financed and operated by the government agency at the local, state or national level. Hospitals provide services at free of cost.

Private Hospitals are owned and operated by churches, corporations, individuals and charitable organizations. Private hospitals are operated on a forprofit- basis.

Military Hospitals provide medical care for the armed forces and their families.

Health Care Services

- Health promotion
  - Prenatal classes
  - Nutrition counselling
  - Family Planning
  - Stress management
- Illness prevention
  - Screening programs (Eg. Hypertension, breast cancer)

   - Immunization
   - Occupational health and safety measures
   - Mental health counseling
   - AIDS control programme.
- Primary care
   - School health units
   - Routine physical examination
   - Follow up for chronic illnesses(eg - Diabetes, Epilepsy)
- Diagnosis
   - Radiological procedure (Eg. CT scans, X ray Studies)
   - Physical examination
   - Laboratory investigations
- Treatment
   - Surgical intervention
   - Laser therapies
   - Pharmacological therapy
- Rehabilitation
   - Cardiovascular programs
   - Sports medicine
   - Mental illness programme

Chapter 2

Hospital and its Environment

Hospitals are institutions, which are mainly designed to care for the sick, injured and the well. The later are usually admitted for physical check up and investigations which cannot be done elsewhere.

In our country most of the government hospitals offer free treatment for people with poor, socio-economic condition, which helps in the alleviations of untold misery. The word hospital is derived from the word "hopes" which means a guest.

This is quite true for a patient leaves his home and comes to the hospital as a guest for brief periods of stay. Even more than a guest he is worried and sick as such he needs more care and attention than a guest would receive. In the hospital the variety of people of all ages, caste and creed with varying degrees of illness are treated.

Besides the patients there are the workers like doctors, nurses, technicians, fourth class servants and other members of the health team. It is important that the nurse understands the peculiar nature of the patient's stay in the hospital and make the physical, mental and social environment conducive to recovery.

TYPES OF HOSPITALS

Hospitals may be owned by private agencies, individual or government. There are general hospitals where all kinds of services are given such as medical, surgical, paediatrics, obstetrics and other kinds of special service. Some hospitals give only one particular type of service according to sex, age and nature of illness, for example, they may be women's, children's and mental hospitals (Psychiatric Hospital).

THE FUNCTIONS OF THE HOSPITAL

The main aim of a hospital is patient care and comfort and the nurse has much to contribute in not only doing her functions, but also in co-ordinating the activities of the health team. Besides the basic functions of a hospital such as care of the sick and injured, diagnosis, treatment and rehabilitative services, many undertake education of doctors, nurses, technicians etc., as an added function. Some hospitals do research work.

There are various departments in a hospital like medical, nursing, pharmacy, and dietary. Every hospital and its departments have own policies and rules, which govern their various activities.

The nurse should acquaint herself with the policies and interpret those connected with the patient's admission, treatment and discharge to the patient's relatives in a simple language. They must be careful and get the guidance of seniors when dealing with accident patients and other patients with legal implications (medico-legal).

MEETING PATIENT'S NEEDS-NURSES' RESPONSIBILITIES

Every woman should learn the art of cleaning; everyone should be able to keep a home clean. Every nurse should know how to keep her ward clean, and this is best learned by practice. A ward head nurse-in-charge is able to train her domestic staff and guide her nurses in ways of cleanliness because she understands methods of cleaning. Germs live in dust and are a source of infection.

Hence, some authorities state that dusting and cleaning should be done by domestic staff and not touched by the nurses. This also means that domestic staff, i.e., ward workers (class IV workers) should not do anything for the patients, e.g., carrying of crockery.

It is necessary that the ward is kept clean so that growth

of germs is inhibited. A nurse should be able to keep her ward clean. However, too much domestic work is not advocated.

Cleaning of Ward

- Unnecessary articles such as crockery should be removed.
- High dusting is done, for ceilings and walls.
- The beds are made so that bits fall to the floor.
- Beds, etc., are pulled out.
- Sweeping is done A tray is prepared for dusting and cleaning
  - Two dusters, one wet, one dry.
  - A bowl of water.
  - A receiver of bits.
  - Metal polish.
  - Furniture polish and dusters.
  - Soap in a dish.

Some method should be chosen, such as following: (The ward cleaning is usually supervised by the nurses).

- Begin at one end, and work round.
- When things are washable they should be dusted with wet and polished with dry duster.
- Dust is wiped into the duster and not flicked on the floor.
- Furniture surfaces are polished with furniture polish and tiled surfaces washed with soap and water.
- Dusting of the lamps depends upon their height, but they must not be forgotten. Dust must be removed from windows and doors. Usually furniture is polished once a week.
- The inside of the lockers are washed once a week.
- The floor is washed by the class IV workers.
- Gusts of wind will disturb dust. It is usual to open the windows on the opposite side from which the wind is blowing whilst dusting is in progress.
- Screens must be dusted.
- Oiling is done periodically. Fluff must be removed from chair legs and screen wheels.

- Washbasins require to be washed with vim powder.

Care of Kitchen

- Food cupboard is cleaned daily. Each article should have a definite place.
- Sinks must not be allowed to become blocked. Waste food should be placed in the rubbish bin and removed daily. The bin should be emptied and cleaned daily.
- Both bucket and rubbish bin should have tightly fitting lids which should be properly replaced.
- Should the sinks become blocked, simple measures may be tried to unblock it. A label should be placed on the sink with "out of use" on it.
- Food must not be left exposed in the kitchen. Milk must always be kept covered.

Care of Linen

- This must be properly stamped with the ward and hospital names so that it is not lost in the laundry or in the ward.
- New articles should be washed before use.
- Torn linen should be put aside for repair.
- Stains should be removed at once before they become fixed.
- Wet articles must not be left in the dirty linen bin.
- Dirty linen should be sent to laundry promptly.
- Linen is carefully sorted, on its return from the laundry and discrepancies reported.
- Stock-taking must be accurate and frequent so that track is kept on lost articles.
- Dirty linen is sorted and account is written when sending to laundry.

Care of Rubber Articles

- All mackintoshes and rubber articles should be washed in warm soapy water, rinsed and carbolised with 1 in 20 carbolic lotion. Dry thoroughly in a cool place and french chalk powder is sprinkled and either rolled or hung up, never folded. Dry heat and hot sun destroy rubber. Sun causes it to blister. Turpentine will do this too.

- Two rubber surfaces should not come together but must be separated. In the case of hot water bottle, the surfaces are separated by air.
- Mackintoshes in the store cupboard should be examined weekly. If the air is moist, the mackintosh may become sticky.
- Kinking the rubber tubing is ruinous.
- Excessive steam causes rubber gloves to become hard.
- Ointments spoil rubber.
- Excessive boiling makes rubber limp and overstretched.
- Rubber articles should be stored in the dark.

Disinfecting the ward Equipments

- Linen and bandages: Receive into a bucket at bedside containing disinfectant lotion-carbolic lotion 1:40. Keep for 4 hours.
- Pus, urine, stools, vomit and sputum are disinfected before disposal in carbolic lotion1: 20 for 2 hrs.
- Immerse receptacles in phenyl lotion 1:20 for 2 hours Rinse them before use.
- Infected furniture and mackintoshes: Mop with carbolic lotion 1:20 before routine cleansing.
- Infected blankets, pillows and mattresses: In most hospitals these are submitted to steam sterilisation e.g. 25 1bs. pressure at 260°F for ½ an hour.
- Crockery and glassware when it is inconvenient to boil: These may be immersed in carbolic lotion 1:20 for 2 hours. Wash thoroughly before use.

Care of the Sanitary Annexe

Care of the Sanitary Annexe is Considered to Important and the Steps are

- This is cleaned thoroughly daily, tidied at frequent intervals and well ventilated.

- Insides and outsides of the sinks are cleaned.
- Bedpans and urinals are washed with hot soapy water.
- Bedpans and urinals are stored in large tanks containing a suitable cheap disinfectant, which is changed daily.
- Ventilated cupboards may be provided for bedpan storage.
- Enamelware is washed daily and stains removed before they become fixed.
- The sanitary annex should have the following: 1) Lavatory brush and mop. 2) A bucket with a tightly fitting lid to receive dressings prior to their removal to the incinerator. 3) Soil linen box.

Care of the Flush out

- This is cleaned daily.
- Frequent flushing is required.
- The lavatory brush is stored in a disinfectant, which is changed daily.

Care of the Bath Room

Walls and floors of bath room should be washed daily.

Stock Taking

- Stock taking is done periodically of all kitchen utensil, cutlery and dressing instruments.
- This ensures the nurses with a sense of responsibility. Stock taking of linen and equipment is taken at definite intervals, e.g. every three months.
- Certain days are allocated for reporting of repairs, losses and breakages.

Hospital Economy

- Economy of time is too often neglected. If a nurse is undecided about the method of carrying out a duty, she should ask for guidance and not waste time in her efforts of trial and error. It is quicker in the long run to do things correctly.

- A nurse should look after her health so that working hours are not lost through illness.
- Daily inventories of important instruments will prevent their loss.

Dressings

- Dressing should be large enough to cover the wound only. Old blankets are used for medical fomentations and not lint. A wide bandage should not be used when a small one will do. Dressing lotions should be carefully measured so that there is no waste.
  - During dressing, the bed-linen is protected by a dressing mackintosh and dressing towel.
  - Taps, lights and gas should be turned off when not in use. Faulty taps must be reported. Kettles sterilizers and saucepans must not be allowed to boil dry, or left on the gas unnecessarily. The kettle should not be filled when a small quantity of hot water is required.
  - Articles must be used for the purpose for which they are made.
  - Medicine and drugs must be accurately used as ordered. Many deteriorate from exposure or evaporation.
  - Soap must not be allowed to stay in water.
  - Disinfectants should not be wasted or used in wrong strengths.
  - Cleaning powders, furniture polish and metal polish should be used sparingly.
  - Torn linen must not be used without mending or it may be torn further and rendered useless.
  - Bed linen should be protected wherever necessary.
  - During meals patient' s wear and bed lines are protected with towels.
  - A small amount of diet should be given to a

patient and a second help if desired and permitted. Excess food should be returned to the main kitchen.

- Although patients should look as nice as possible, it must be remembered that laundering involves wear and tear and is very expensive.
- Crockery must be handled carefully and not allowed to chip or crack.
- Nurses should be taught the prices of articles, lotions etc.
- False economy is stupid and even criminal on occasions.
- Nurses must remember that hospitals are maintained with the public's money. The people can often ill afford their contributions.
- Each ward is assessed separately and list of expenses sent round to the wards. They impress the nursing staff and encourage economy.

Admission, Observation, Charting, Feeding and Discharge Admission of the Patient

The entrance of a patient into a health care agency such as a hospital or a private clinic is termed as admission. A patient enters the hospital by himself or he may be brought to the hospital by his relatives, friends, neighbours or others. Mentally ill patients, persons who have tried to commit suicide and accident patients are admitted through a legal process.

All ill person enters the hospital to get his disorder cured whereas a healthy individual gets admitted into a hospital for a day or two for investigations and observations and in order to find out whether he is suffering from any illness which has not been manifested by any external signs and symptoms. Patients who have become seriously ill suddenly, come to the hospital without having had any time to settle their family and work affairs.

Hence, they are not only worried and anxious about their illness, but also are upset about various other problems affecting their family.

Nurses must understand their physical and mental problems and be very kind and understanding.

Need for Good Reception of the Patient

A nurse has an important role to play in the reception of the patient to the hospital. The following are the purposes of this procedure.

- To prepare the patient both physically and mentally for his stay in the hospital.
- To help the patient to be comfortable and to provide him with a clean and safe environment.
- To give a good impression of the hospital and its services so that the patient will fully co-operate with the treatment and nursing care.

A patient may be coming to hospital for the first time. He leaves his familiar home surrounding and his loved ones and comes to an unknown place and to unknown people. Any change in human life is anxiety producing and is viewed with fear. Added to this, his physical condition gives him fear and anxiety. Hence, it is the nurse's duty to receive the patient, kindly sympathetically and with an understanding of his illness.

If he is admitted, he is given a diet sheet and sent to the ward. If he is too ill and needs immediate attention he is given emergency treatment and then transported to the ward. As soon as the patient comes to the ward, receive him, his relatives and his friends as if you are receiving your guests into your home. Ask them to be seated while you prepare the bed ready for the patient.

If the patient is in a serious condition, the ward nurse is informed in advance about the arrival of the patient, so that the patient does not have to wait till the bed is made ready.

Need for Orientation to Place and People

Inform the patient and his relatives about the hospital routine, the hospital rules, the general set up of the ward and the personnel working in the ward. Inform the patient's relatives about the time of visiting hours and supply them with visiting passes. If the patient is seriously ill, give the relative a special pass so that he will be able to stay with the patient in the hospital.

Need for Admission Assessment

Do a good assessment of his physical condition in order to plan his care. If his physical state needs immediate treatment report to physician and prepare your patient for physical examination and carry out the treatment, which the physician prescribes after the physical examination.

Need for Safeguarding Patient's Personal Belongings

It is always good policy to discourage patients to keep valuable things and money with them. Send the valuables home through relatives. If he does not have anyone with him, enter the description of items in the register and send the valuables to the office for safe custody. Get the patient's signature or thumb impression in the register. However, inform the patient that he will get back his valuables on discharge.

It is important that you take care of the patient's clothing. You should see that the clothing are cleaned and stored away with proper label or send them home for a fresh set of clean clothes. However, encourage, patients to use hospital clothing. If a patient is suffering from infectious disease, see that the clothing are disinfected and cleaned before they are sent home or stored away.

Need for Personal Hygiene

As a nurse it is important that you attend the personal hygiene of the patient on admission. If the patient is able to have a bath in the bathroom, he can be given a bath. If he is unable to walk, you can give him a bed-bath. You should carry out other aspects of your patient's personal hygiene such as care of hair, mouth and nails.

Especially in our country, the patients who are ignorant and illiterate do not see to their personal hygiene when they become sick. So when a patient comes to the hospital, this need has to be attended to on his admission. During the process of cleaning your patient, you get an opportunity to examine and observe him thoroughly and talk to him so that you will be able to know about his physical and mental condition.

Observation of the Patient

Webster's dictionary defines observation as "the act or power of noticing". Nurses are with the patients throughout day and night. Your report of observation is very valuable in helping the physician to arrive at proper diagnosis and treatment. The essence of good nursing depends largely on intelligent observation. It is through observation you notice your patients' deviations from normal condition.

Your observation and prompt actions may help patients from getting into serious complications such as hemorrhage and other similar problems. Your plan of nursing care also depends upon good observation. Good observation depends on your intelligence and knowledge. Skill in observation is acquired through careful training in using your senses namely, seeing, hearing, touching and smelling.

It is through the sense of seeing you observe whether the patient is walking with difficulty, whether he is in pain and whether he has any other visible problems.

From hearing the sound of his breathing you will able to understand whether the patient is having difficulty in breathing. Touching the patient reveals whether his body temperature is raised above normal or whether the skin is of normal texture or not.

Your sense of smell tells you the nature of discharge from wounds and body cavities. Observation is a continuous process as a patient's condition is never static. It changes continuously. These changes are noticed through careful observation. A nurse's observation includes not only the physical condition of the patient, but also his psychological aspects. Your observation becomes meaningful when it is accompanied by questioning.

To come to clear interpretations of your observations, you have to question you patient so that you will be able to find out the problems experienced by the patient. Through observation you identify the objective symptoms of your patient. Changes in colour of the skin, pulse, respiration, discharges from body cavities and changes in speech are some of the examples of objective symptoms.

Pain nausea, fear, anxiety, dizziness and itching are identified by questioning the patient. These are examples of subjective symptoms.

Certain symptoms cannot be identified by observation or questioning. For example, some special techniques are needed to note changes in temperature, pulse respiration and blood pressure; X-rays and laboratory tests are used for finding out changes in structure and functions of various systems of the human body.

- Physicians use methods such as inspection, palpation, percussion and auscultation for observation of patient's condition.
- Inspection is man's observing with eye.
- Palpation is the art of feeling with the hand.
- Percussion and auscultation depend on the production of sound.
- Percussion is tapping an area to produce sounds.
- Auscultation is listening to sounds within the body with a stethoscope. It is the art of hearing the heart sound, bowel movement etc.
- *Olfaction*: Sense of smell. (odour)

Specific observations When a patient comes to the hospital or clinic, do an overall observation of the patient, note down his problems, report to the senior nurse and write your observations in the nurse's record sheet. Use the following as a guide for your observation and for estimation of your patient's condition.

The General Structure of the Body

- Whether he is obese, malnourished, acutely ill or chronically ill.
- Whether he is weak and unable to walk or walks with aid

- Whether he is in pain
- Note the colour of the skin-pale, jaundiced.

Mental Status and level of Consciousness

- Whether the patient is cheerful or depressed, anxious and worried, irritate, afraid or sad.
- Whether oriented to place, person and time.
- Whether fully conscious, drowsy or comatose.

Hair and Scalp

- Whether the hair is clean, thick, thin, matted, dirty or coarse.
- Whether there is any lesion, dandruff, pediculi or nits on the scalp.

Eyes

- Whether the eyes are protruding, sunken or crossed. Whether the colour is abnormal - Reddish or yellow.
- Whether there is swelling, discharge, abnormal watering, pain, burning, itching, photophobia or headache.
- Whether the vision is normal or poor.
- Whether the patient uses glasses.

Face

- Whether the face is pale, flushed or jaundiced.
- Whether there is swelling, ulcers, rashes or injuries.
- Whether his checks are swollen or sunken.

Mouth

- Whether his breath smells of drugs or alcohol or has a bad smell.
- Whether the gum is inflamed, swollen, bleeding or uncrated.
- Whether the lips are cyanotic, dry swollen, cracked or ulcerated.
- Whether the teeth are loose, broken, artificial or irregularly arranged

- Whether he has any toothache.
- Whether the taste is impaired or disturbed
- Whether the tongue is dry, cracked, coated, inflamed, ulcerated, blistered, fissured or swollen.

Throat

- Whether the patient has any ulcer, inflammation or pain. Whether he has any difficulty in swallowing.

Speech

- Whether the speech is absent
- Whether he has any difficulty in speech-stammering or incoherent.
- Whether the voice is hoarse or weak.

Nose

- Whether there is any deformity, swelling or discharge of mucous, blood or pus.
- Whether the sense of smell is present or absent.

Ears

- Whether he is able to hear or not
- Whether there is collection of wax in the ear.
- Whether the patient experiences any ringing or buzzing sounds, dizziness, itching or pricking.

Neck

- Whether the patient has pain and difficulty in moving the neck.
- Whether there is any swelling or distended vein.

Chest

- Whether the patient suffers from cough
- Whether the sputum is of abnormal colour or quantity
- Whether the breathing is laboured or normal.

Breast

- Whether there are any abnormalities in the shape and size.

- Whether there are any lumps or discharge from the nipples.

Abdomen

- Whether it is soft, tender, distended, hard, swollen, flabby or protruding.
- Whether he has any nausea, vomiting or pain.
- Whether his appetite is normal or not.

Extremities

- Whether the nails are broken or brittle
- Whether there is clubbing of fingertips, tremors of hands, swelling of extremities, pain in the joints or any other abnormality.

Skin

- Whether there are any sores, wounds, rashes or scales.
- Whether the skin is dry, moist, hot, cold or clammy.

Excretions and Discharges

- Whether the colour, consistency, amount, odour, and characteristics of stools, urine, sputum, perspiration, vomitus and vaginal discharge are normal or abnormal.
- Whether patient gets any pain or any other discomfort during excretion.

CHARTING

The nurses are required to report and record their observations. She reports her findings to the professional nurse and to the physician. Recording of the observations is called charting. The nurses should chart their observations correctly. All chartings should be brief, concise, account and complete. Charting helps physicians, nurses and others to understand the condition and progress of the patient. The chart is also used for legal procedures and research.

A patient's chart includes records maintained by

physicians and nurses. A nurse should be able to maintain records related to nursing and she should be able to understand the notes made by physicians and others.

Safety and Comfortable Environment

The environment in which the patient is placed should be comfortable and safe and it should contribute to his well being and should not retard his recovery.

Safety and Comfort Measures

Safety means protection from possible injury. Many factors contribute towards the safety of patients in the hospital. The hospital buildings should be structurally sound for ensuring safety for patients with physical limitations such as, blind, aged or handicapped.

The nursing personnel must be safety conscious and they should take all efforts to prevent accidents in the hospital. She should report all accidents promptly and take measures to prevent them from happening again. A register should be maintained for recording accidents.

Mechanical Devices for Comfort Measures

To hospitals use many mechanical devices for ensuring safety/patients.

- Bed bars (side rails) are used to prevent patients from falling out of bed. Patients who requires this safety measure are post operative patients, unconscious, semi-conscious mentally disturbed, sedated, blind or children or very old patients.
- Back rest: These are usually made of metals. These are used to support the back of the patient in upright position.
- Over bed table: The table such as the cardiac table is placed in front of the patient and the top of the table is adjusted to the desired height. As pillow is arranged on the top of the table so that the patient can lean forward on it for support.

When he wants to take food, read or write.

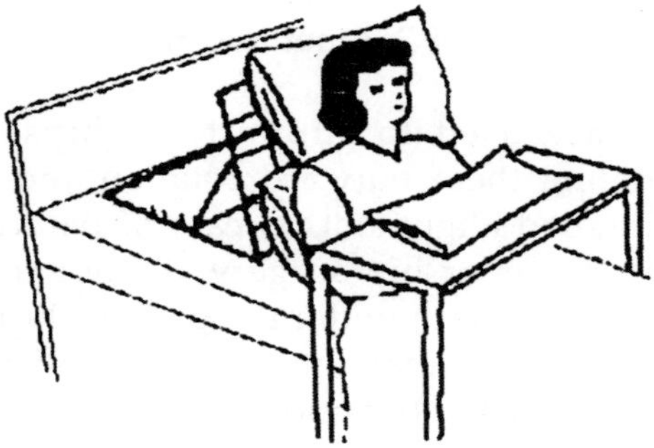

Fig. A patient resting with back rest and over bed table (Cardiac table)

- Foot-boards: (Foot-rests): These are made of wood and are L shaped, so that one end can be slipped under the mattress to hold the other end in a firm upright position. The patient is placed in supine position to rest the bottoms of the feet flat against the surface of the foot-board (covered with sheet). These are used to prevent foot drop by maintaining good alignment.
- Sand-bags: These are canvas, rubber or plastic bags filled with sand and are 1,5 and 10 lbs in weight. These are used to immobilize the body part, placing them snugly next to the part. Eg. On either side of the feet to maintain the position of the feet on the footboard, immobilize the fractured limb.
- Blocks (shock blocks): These are made of wood, may be high or low. These are placed under the foot of the bed for various reasons. Eg. surgical shock, traction and postural drainage. This may be placed under the head of bed to promote drainage and improve cerebral circulation.
- Hand rolls: These are made of cloth that is rolled into a cylinder about 4-5 inches long and 2-3 inches in diameter and stuffed firmly. These are used to keep the fingers form being held in a tight fist leading to flexion contracture in patients who are unable to move the hands due to paralysis, injury or disease

- Thigh rolls: These are made by folding a sheet to a desired length of 2-3 feet and then rolled into a tight cylinder.
  These are used to support the hips and thighs, preventing them outward rotation and keeping the feet in good alignment, in case of paralysis, fracture of the femur or hip surgery. To use the roll, place the lose end (flap) under the patients hips and thighs with the role under the flap end and then tucking snugly along the hip and thigh
- Cradle: These are mostly semicircular in shape, made of wood or metal.
  These are used to prevent the weight of top bedclothes on patient' s feet and toes. To use the cradle, Place it over the bottom bedclothes and the top bedclothes are then brought over the cradle. These are used for patients affected by burns.
- Restraints are devices used to prevent agitated patients, persons who get out of bed at night in their sleep and small children, from falling out of bed.
- Wire mesh for windows and doors are fixed to prevent insects.

COMMON HAZARDS

- Patients should be safeguarded from fire accidents and from careless application of heat. Fire accidents occur mainly due to allowing patients to smoke in bed, use of faulty electric appliances, and careless use of oxygen cylinders.
- Patient may get injured from careless application of hot water bags, electric pads and application of medications on the skin.
- Poisonous drugs should be kept under lock and key with specific red label.
- Patients may come to harm through bacteriological sources, insects and rodents. Food and water should be made safe for consumption. Insects and rodents should be eliminated.

COMFORT

Comfort is a sense of mental and physical well being.

Physical Comfort

Physical comfort gets affected due to a dirty and wet bed and lack of body alignment. High temperature and humidity, poor ventilation, too much noise, unpleasant odours and glaring lighting make the patient uncomfortable.

To promote comfort for the patients, certain mechanical devices can be used. Pillows can be used for giving support for the various part of the body. Sometimes-patient feels comfortable in a propped up position. In a hospital, a backrest is provided for the patient to keep him in a sitting position. For relaxation of abdominal muscles, when patients are in pain or after an abdominal operation, knees can be kept flexed by means of a knee rest.

A pillow or a blanket or sheet rolled as a pillow can be improvised as a knee rest. Patients should not be kept with flexed knees for a long period. His circulation may get affected. Hence his position is changed frequently. For supporting feet and for preventing foot drop, foot rests are used. This device keeps the feet at right angles to the leg and prevents deformities. Foot-rest can be improvised with sand bags. Other devices used as comfort measures are air rings or cotton rings and air cushions to prevent pressure ulcer.

Mental Comfort

Mental comfort is provided for the patient by eliminating his fear, anxiety and worry. He should receive sympathy and consideration from the nursing and medical staff. His relatives should avoid unpleasant news to him while he is in the hospital. Meeting his spiritual needs may help to give him mental peace and comfort.

FEEDING OF PATIENTS

Preparing and serving of patient. Meals should be accurately prepared, according to the requirements of the individual patient and his disease. Great care should be taken and be kept away from the patient to avoid spilling. Meals should be attractively served. The plate should be clean on both surfaces. A nicely prepared, well cooked food improves appetite. The patient must be placed in the most suitable position and the plate is conveniently placed. A towel must be placed around his neck so that it gives maximum protection to the patient and bedclothes. Hot food should be given if permitted.

Spoon Feeding

This is often used for the feeding of children and patients who cannot feed themselves. The spoon should be of suitable size and time should be allowed for the mastication. The nurse should appear unhurried. It is usual for the nurse to stand on the right side of the patient but exceptions occur. Help the patient to take their feeds who are unable to feed themselves and everything possible must be done to alleviate the feeling of helplessness.

Children with harelips and cleft palate are mostly spoon fed; sometimes a special spoon is used and after operation, a sterile spoon is used. The child should be well supported and the spoon placed well to the back of the mouth. After operations for harelip or cleft palate, great care should be taken to prevent the spoon from touching the suture lines.

Feeding with a Feeding Cup

The feeder (feeding cup) must be perfectly clean, especially the spout and under the over hanging half-lid. It should be placed on a saucer with a spoon, and carried to the bed side on a tray which is covered with a tray cloth. Spread a towel around the patient' s neck. The feed should not be too hot. The nurse' s left arm should be placed under the pillow to raise the patient' s head and the spout of the feeder placed between his lips.

The patient should be taught to place his tongue over the spout tip when requiring a rest, or to make a sign to the nurse. In some instances, feeding is made more easy if a piece of rubber tubing is attached to the spout of the feeder, this should be carefully washed and boiled at least once daily. In some cases both feeder and rubber spout are boiled before and after each feed. A special brush is provided for the cleaning of spouted feeders. At the end of the meal, the patient' s mouth should be dried, in some cases the mouth may require cleaning before and after the meal.

DISCHARGING THE PATIENT

Discharge is a preparation of a patient and discharge records to leave the hospital.

Purpose

- To ensure continuity of care to the patient after discharge
- To assist the patient in discharge process

Guidelines

The patient are discharged from the hospital in one of the following ways

Discharge to Home

The discharge to home or another hospital or another unit within the hospital is initiated by the doctor who advises the patient that he is well enough to leave the hospital or requires treatment in another unit within the hospital or in an another hospital.

Discharge to Another Hospital or Another Unit Within the Hospital (referral)

When a patient or family is not satisfied with the treatment or care given and wants to leave the hospital against the medical advice, in such cases the patient or the relative is asked to sign a statement that he is going or taking the patient on his own will and responsibility.

Discharge Against Medical Advice (AMA)

Patient leaves the hospital against the medical officer' s advice. When a patient escapes from the hospital without the knowledge of the hospital staff and without signing the said statement he is treated as absconded in the records.

NURSES RESPONSIBILITY

- Inform the patient and the relatives a day or two before the discharge
- Get the discharge slip prepared after checking the vital signs and examining the patient.
- The nurses should see that the patients personnel hygiene is maintained, he is dressed in home clothes and has taken meals.
- Hand over the patient's belongings and any valuables, which have been kept safely, to the patient or the relative under proper receipt.
- Complete the unit admission and discharge registers, case sheet and other records.
- Hand over the case sheet and other records to medical record department under proper receipt.
- Inform the hospital authorities about the discharge if the patient is medico-legal.
- Hand over the discharge slip to the patient or relative and explain about
  - The treatment and the diet to be taken at home
  - Follow-up visits and inform to bring the discharge slip on every visits
  - Any special advices pertaining to condition
- See that the patient receives all the medicines as per discharge slip.
- Check the hospital things before the patient leaves the ward.
- Place the patient in the wheel chair or stretcher according to the patient' s condition until he leaves the hospital.
- Immediately after the patient leaves, reorganise the patient unit.

Chapter 3

Infection Control

Good health depends in part on a safe environment. Practices that control and prevent transmission of infection help to protect patients and health workers from disease. Patients admitted in hospitals are at risk for acquiring infections because of lower resistance to infections microorganisms, increased exposure to number and types of disease causing microorganisms and invasive procedures.

Health care workers can protect themselves from contact with infectious material or exposure to communicable diseases by having knowledge of the infectious process and appropriate barrier protection Hepatitis B.

AIDS and tuberculosis have caused a greater emphasis on infection control techniques. Knowledge of microbiology is an essential component in nursing for practicing disinfections and sterilization to eliminate pathogenic microbes causing infectious disease. Microbiology is a study of life process of the smallest living organisms (microbes). Microbes are so small that they can be seen only with the aid of a microscope.

CLASSIFICATION OF MICRO ORGANISMS

Microorganisms are classified as follows:

- *Virus:* Viruses are very minute living organisms, which can pass through bacterial filters and can be seen only under electron microscope.
- *Bacteria:* Bacteria are heterogenous and belong to both animal and plant kingdom.
- *Streptococci:* They are round shaped organisms

arranged in chain. They are gram positive, non-motile, highly pathogenic and do not grow in ordinary media. They grow in blood and serum media.

- *Staphylococci:* Staphylococci are arranged in clusters like grapes. They are gram positive and violet in colour when stained.
  They are non-motile and non-spore forming organisms. There are two types of pathogenic staphylococci (a) Staphylococcus albus and (b) Staphyloccus aureus.
- *Diplococci:* Diplococci are arranged in pairs and they are gram-negative organisms. Examples of diplococci are Neisseria gonococci and Neisseria meningococci. They grow in special culture media of heated blood.
- *Pneumococci:* Pneumococci are also arranged in pairs. They are gram-positive and found in nasopharynx.
- *Bacillus:* Bacilli are rod shaped organisms. These are gram positive and gram-negative organisms. Grampositive bacilli are Corynebacterium diptheriae, clostridium tetani and bacillus anthracis and mycobacterium tuberculosis.
- *Clostridium Tetani:* Clostridium tetani or bacillus tetani are rod shaped spore forming organisms. Mostly they are found in the intestinal tract of man and animals. They are also present in soil.
- *Bacillus anthracis:* Bacilli anthracis are large rods with spores. They are found in animal hairs, wool, soil, water and dust.
- *Escherichia coli:* These are small rod shaped organisms, sometimes motile and sometimes encapsulated. They are found in the intestinal tracts of man and animals and they are non-pathogenic.
- *Salmonella:* Like E.coli, Salmonella also are small, motile and rod shaped bacilli.
- *Vibrio:* Vibrio are cama shaped, motile, gram negative and non-spore forming organisms
- *Rickettsiae:* Rickettsiae are larger than virus and

smaller than bacteria in size. They are variously shaped like minute rods or spheres.

- *Virus:* Viruses are the lowest form of living creatures, which are capable of reproduction. They are ultra microscopic structures and are not visible in ordinary microscope. They are visible only in electron microscope.

COMMON VIRAL AND DISEASES OF MAN

Organisms	Mode of entry	Disease
Virus variola	Inhalation	Small pox
Influenza	Inhalation	Epidemic influenza
Virus varicella	Mouth	Mumps
Virus rubella	Inhalation	Measles
Virus hepatitis Virus A Virus B	 Ingestion Inoculation	 Infective hepatitis Serum hepatitis
Polio virus	Ingestion	Poliomyelitis
Human Immuno Defeciency Virus	Inoculation, transplacental Sexual contact	Acquired Immuno Deficiency Syndrome

METHODS USED FOR IDENTIFICATION OF MICROBES

Microbes are considered as unseen enemies of man. They can be seen only under microscope. To identify the specific microbes, the following methods are done. Smear, fixing, hanging drop preparation, staining, culture, animal inoculation, serological tests.

Microscope

Microscope is the instrument, which is used to magnify objects, and structure, which are too small to see by the naked eye. Since the science of microbiology is concerned with the microorganisms, we can appreciate that microscope is the most essential piece of equipment in the laboratory to identify bacteria. There are varieties of microscopes of which three are most important.

- The compound optical microscope, which is used for routine bacteriological examinations.
- The dark field microscope, which is used to identify spirochaetes, e.g. trepenoma pallidum
- The electron microscope is the most powerful microscope used to maginify the object by 100,000 times.

This is used in the identification of viruses.

- *Smear:* Place a drop of specimen, which is to be examined, on the middle of a slide. Place a drop of distilled water (Water is needed only for solid specimen, e.g. motion) with a sterile loop, and spread the specimen uniformly on the slide. This kind of examination is known as direct microscopic examination.
- *Fixing:* Fix the smear by flaming the slide. Flaming is done by passing the slide on a flame for three or four times. Fixing can also be done by using chemicals such as formalin, methyl alcohol, mercuric chloride.
- *Hanging Drop Preparation:* It is often used to determine whether the bacteria are motile or non-motile. Hanging drop preparation aids in studying the organisms in living state. Human Immuno Deficiency Virus: It is identified by ELISA and Westernblot tests.

TYPES OF SPECIMEN COLLECTED

- *Swabs:* It is usually collected in a sterile test tube. Care should be taken so as to prevent contaminations of specimen.
- *Throat swab for cultures:* These should be taken only with a view of the throat, in a good light and using a tongue depressor. Materials should be taken only from the infected area.
- *Sputum:* It should be collected in a sterile container having wide mouth. Sputum should be collected directly after a cough and sent immediately to the laboratory.

- *Urine:* Urine specimen for chemical and microscopic examinations can be collected in a clean container or test tube, but for culture it should be collected in a sterile test tube.
- *Faeces:* Fresh stools should be collected for bacteriological examination.
- *Blood:* It should be collected in a sterile container. The nurse should assist while collecting other specimens like cerebro spinal fluid.
  Etc. When assisting the physician, she should adopt aseptic precautions so as to avoid contamination of specimen.

TERMINOLOGIES

- *Pathogens:* Microorganisms, those are capable of producing disease.
- *Asymptamatic infection:* If the microorganisms fail to cause serious injuries to cells or tissues and patient is symptom free of the particular disease.
- *Disease:* The pathogens multiply and cause an alteration is normal tissues and manifest with signs and symptoms.
- *Communicable disease:* If the infectious disease can be transmitted directly from one person to another, it is known as communicable disease or contagious disease.
- *Disinfection:* It is a process by which pathogenic organisms are killed by physical and chemical agents.
- *Disinfectant:* It is a chemical substance, which kills the pathogenic microorganisms or organisms capable of giving rise to infection, e.g. Iodine, phenyl, carbolic acid.
- *Antiseptic:* It is a chemical substance which inhibits the growth of microorganisms and do not kill the organisms (e.g.) dettol.
- *Detergents:* Detergent increases the cleaning power of water and leaves no film or scum. Some are used only for cleaning without any bacteriocidal action.

- *Bacteriostasis:* It is a process of inhibiting the growth of bacteria (e.g.) Freezing and drying.
- *Bacteriocide:* It is a substance, which kills microorganisms.
- *Sepsis:* It is a term used for the presence of pathogenic organisms.
- *Inflammation:* The body' s cellular response to injury or infection is inflammation.
- *Antigen:* Remnents of the micro organisms that trigger the immune response. Antigens are usually composed of proteins.
- *Antibodies:* Antibodies are large protein molecules. Antibodies are immunoglobulins, which are synthesized and secreted by the plasma cells when an antigen enters the body, to neutralise the antigen. Types of immunoglobulin lgA. Ig D, Ig E, Ig G and Ig M, The most abundant circulating antibody in lgG.
- *Sterilisation:* Strelisation is defined as the process by which an article, surface, or medium is free of all microorganisne' sms, either in the vegetative or spore state.
- Chemotherapy It is the treatment of disease by means of chemicals, which are known as chemotherapeutic agents (e.g.) Sulphonamides. Destruction or inhibition of growth of organisms depends upon the concentration of chemotherapeutic agents.
- *Antibiotics:* These are drugs used to kill the organisms (e.g.) Pencillin.
- *Local infection:* An infection that is localized within a particular part or a single organ. Proper care controls spread.
- *Systemic infection:* An infection that affects the entire body. It can become fatal.

Infection Process

Development of an infection occurs in a cycle that depends on the following elements.

- An infection agent or pathogen

- Source for pathogen growth (A reservoir)
- A portal of exit from the reservoir
- A mode of transmission
- A portal of entry to a host
- A susceptible host

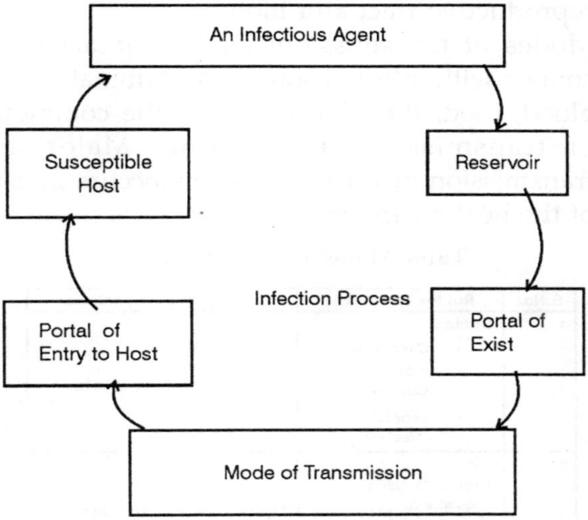

Fig. Chain of infection

An infection will develop if this chain remains intact. Nurses use infection prevention and control practices to break the chain so that infection will not develop.

Infectious Agent

Microorganisms include bacteria, viruses, fungi and protozoa. They are the common infectious agents. The potential for microorganisms or parasites to cause disease depends on the following factors:

- Sufficient number of organisms
- Virulence or ability to produce disease
- Ability to enter and survive to the host
- Susceptibility of host.

Reservoir

A reservoir is where a pathogen can survive. Skin of

patients, carriers, animals, food, water insects, and inanimate objects are common reservoirs of infection.

- Portal of exist Microorganisms can enter through a variety of sites such as skin and mucous membrane, respiratory tract, urinary tract, gastrointestinal tract, reproductive tract and blood.
- Modes of transmission: Direct contact or indirect contact with infected source, contaminated air, water, blood, food, flies, mosquito are the common modes of transmission to infection. Major mode of transmission of microorganisms occurs in the hands of the health care providers.

Table Modes of transmission

S.No.	Routes and means	Examples of Organisms
1	**Contact** a. Direct Contact b. Indirect Contact c. Droplet Infection	Hepatitis A Virus Hepatitis B Virus Measles Virus, Rubella Virus
2	**Air** Droplet Nuclei (Residue or Evaporated Droplets Suspended in air)	Mycobacterium Tuberculosis
3	**Vehicles** a. Contaminated Items Water	Vibrio Cholera Hepatitis C.

- Portal of entry: Organisms can enter the body through skin, mucus membranes, respiratory tract, gastro intestinal tract, reproductive tract and blood.
- Susceptible host Whether a person acquires an infection depends on susceptibility to an infectious agent. Susceptibility depends on the individual degree of resistance to a pathogen. The suscepti-bility of host depends upon the virulence of micro-organisms and immune status of the host.

COURSE OF INFECTION BY STAGE

- *Incubation Period*: Interval between entrance of pathogen into body and appearance of first symptoms. eg. chickenpox 2-3 weeks. common cold 1-2 days mumps 18 days

- *Prodromal Stage*: Interval from onset of non-specific signs and symptoms (malaise, low-grade fever, fatigue) to more specific symptoms. During this time, microorganisms grow and multiply and patient is more capable of spreading disease to others.
- *Illness Stage*: Interval when patient manifests signs and symptoms specific to a particular disease. The severity of patient' s illness depends on the extent of infection, the pathogenicity of the micro-organisms and susceptibility of individuals.
- *Convalescence*: Interval when acute symptoms of infection disappear until the individual regain his normal health.Length of recovery depends on severity of infection and patient' s general health status. Recovery may take several days to months.
- *Defences Against Infection*:
  - The body has normal defenses against infection.
  - Normal body flora that reside inside and outside of the body protect a person from several pathogens
  - The inflammatory response is a protective vascular and cellular reaction that neutralizes pathogens and repairs body cells.
  - Each organ system has defence mechanism that defense against exposure to infectious micro organisms.

Nosocomial Infection: Nosocomial infections are infections that are acquired by a patient due to delivery of health care services.Most nosocomial infections are transmitted by health care workers.

- *Iatrogenic Infections*: Iatrogenic infections are a type of nosocomial infection resulting from a diagnostic or therapeutic procedure. (eg) urinary tract infection that develops after catheter insertion. Nosocomial infections may be exogenous infection or endogenous infection.

- *Exogenous Infection*: Exogenous infection arises from microorganisms external to the individual, which do not exist as normal flora.
  Eg. Salmonella typhi-Typhoid fever Clostridium tetani-Tetanus.
- *Endogenous Infection*: Endogenous infection occurs when part of the patients flora becomes altered (virulent) and also increase in number Eg. Streptococci, Enterococci

MECHANICAL

- *Scrubbing*: Hand washing is one of the important procedures of a nurse in order to control and prevent self-infection as well as cross infection. Scrubbing and washing the hands with soap and water removes the organisms mechanically.
- *Filtration*: In laboratories fluids are sterilized by filtration. The process of filtration aids in retaining certain bacteria.
- *Sedimentation*: It is used in the purification of water. By this method the suspending materials together with bacteria settles down in the bottom of liquid.

PHYSICAL METHODS

- *Moist Heat*: Boiling - Boiling at 100°C for 3 to 5 minutes kills microorganisms except spore bearing organisms such as bacillus tetani. There are certain rules to be observed while boiling.
  - Scrub and clean the articles to remove organic matter, which will coagulate around the organisms and protect them.
  - Articles except the glass should be put at the boiling point of water (great care should be taken for glass articles, and they should be wrapped with cloth and put in cold water and then brought to boil).
  - Articles should be well covered by the water and boiled for the required length of time.

Steam under Pressure

Spore bearing organisms are killed by steam under pressure. Autoclave is an apparatus used for sterilization of articles by steam under pressure. In this, the steam is allowed to circulate in a closed container and it is compressed and thereby raises the temperature above the boiling point of water (121°C).

In this method the articles are sterilized under 15 pounds pressure of steam for 15 to 20 minutes. Materials sterilized by autoclaving method are dressings, gloves, linen, syringes, certain instruments and culture medias.

PASTEURIZATION

Pasteurization is a method of sterilizing milk. Milk is heated to a temperature of 60°C for half an hour and rapidly cooled to 13°C. This aids in destroying all pathogenic organisms and reduces acid-producing organisms and thus prevents souring of milk.

Dry Heat Baking

This method of sterilization is used in sterilizing glassware, syringes, needles, culture tubes and medias. Most of the vegetative forms of bacteria are killed. Spores need to be heated for 1 to 2 hours. The apparatus used for baking is known as "hot air oven". Incineration: In order to destroy all organisms, infected wound dressings, contaminated materials, garbage and other hospital wastages etc are burnt by incineration. The apparatus used for this complete burning is incinerator. Flaming: This is used in sterilizing platinum loops in laboratory and also in sterilizing needles and instruments. This aids in killing organisms.

Sunlight

The ultra-violet rays from sunlight have the effect of destroying a large number of bacteria. Blankets, pillows, mattress are disinfected by sunlight. Care should be taken to turn the articles often to kill the microorganisms on both surfaces.

Low Temp Erature

Cold has the effect of decreasing or completely stopping the growth of bacteria. Constant freezing will destroy bacteria.

Chemical Methods

Certain chemicals are used in disinfection of articles like thermometer and also the disinfection of floor and decontamination of infected linen etc.

Principles to be Observed

- All articles contaminated with blood, faeces, pus, sputum, or other substances must be rinsed with cold water to prevent coagulation of protein material.
- Use soap and water for cleaning the instruments and use a brush whenever necessary.
- Allow sufficient time for articles to be disinfected or sterilized by physical or chemical agents.
- It is important to select the right disinfectant, the right strength and the right time.
- Use the right procedure to render instruments and other articles safe for further use in order to prevent the spread of infection.

Chemical Substances, which are Commonly Used

- *Dettol:* This is widely used chemical for sterilization of instruments, thermometer etc.
  It is non-poisonous and non-irritant to the skin. 5 to 50per cent solution is used for dressings and wound irrigation.
- *Savlon:* 1:30 savlon solution is used to destroy or kill vegetative bacteria.
- *Chloride of lime(Bleaching powder):* This is used for disinfection of drinking water, stools, urine, sputum. As it decomposes quickly when exposed to air. Solutions must be made fresh for each use.
- *Formalin:* A 40 per cent solution is used to disinfect faeces, urine and sputum. It is not used for the skin and tissues, as it is an irritant.

- *Tincture of Iodine:* 1-2 per cent iodine is used for cleaning skin and treating injuries to the skin.
- *Hydrogen peroxide:* 1-5 per cent of solution is used in cleaning wounds and to remove pus from infected ears. Hydrogen peroxide is also used to clean the mouth. It is an oxidizing agent.
- *Potassium permanganate:* It is an oxidizing agent used for cleaning the mouth 1:1000 strength. It is also used for irrigation of wounds.
- *Carbolic acid (Phenol):* It is a good disinfectant for faeces, pus, blood and sputum. It is a skin irritant and a poison. Dissolves easily in hot water. For thermometers 1:20 solution for a duration of 10 minutes. 9) Lysol: This is a phenol or chlorasol preparation mixed with soap. It is less poisonous than a carbolic acid but has a greater bacteriocidal action. 2 per cent solution for 6-8 hours is used for disinfecting linen.
- Ethyl alcohol 70per cent is effective for skin disinfection. Certain gases like formaldehyde and gluteral-dehyde are used in disinfection of rooms.

Factors Influencing the Immune Status of Individuals Inherent

- *Racial*: Some races are susceptible or immune to certain diseases. For example, Hebrews are more resistant to tuberculosis than other people.
- *Species*: Some of the species of animals have resistance to certain diseases e.g. lower animals never get measles or typhoid fever while man is susceptible to get these diseases. Birds do not get infection with certain kind of tubercle bacilli, which affects cattle or man.
- *Individual*: some people have a strong natural resistance or immunity to certain diseases. This is known as individual immunity.

Types of Immunity:

- Natural immunity: Natural immunity results after acquiring certain diseases like measles, and usually lasts a life time.

- Artificial immunity: Artificial immunity follows the receipt of a vaccine such as polio vaccine.
- Active immunity: Non-virulent microorganisms are injected as antigens and the body produces antibodies against the antigen.
- Passive immunity: Immunoglobulins or antibodies are injected as a vaccine to neutralize to antigen.
- Acquired immunity: Acquired immunity may be natural or artificial.

Acquired Artificial Immunity: Immunity which, is acquired artificially by introducing vaccine and toxoid (active) and serum (passive) is known as acquired artificial immunity.

Acquired Natural Immunity: People who suffered from disease will have immunity against that particular disease e.g. small pox. This is known as acquired natural active immunity.

Acquired Natural Passive Immunity: The child gets antibodies from its mother through placenta and breast milk and has immunity for sometime against certain diseases.

Types of Immunisation

Active Immunization

It implies administration of antigenic preparation in order to stimulate production of antibodies within the tissues of the individual. This is known as active immunity. The material used for producing active immunity are vaccines (e.g.) BCG vaccine.

Passive Immunization

Sera containing specific antibodies are directly injected to produce passive immunity. Eg. Anti-toxin sera in diphtheria (prepared from horse serum) and tetanus immunoglobulins. Vaccines may consist of: a. Live, virulent organism in sub lethal doses (e.g.) cholera vaccine, anti-rabies vaccine. b. Live attenuated organisms-e.g. vaccine for small pox, tuberculosis (BCG) and yellow fever. c. Dead organisms e.g. vaccines of typhoid, cholera and plague. d. Toxins of organisms, such as toxoids - e.g. vaccines for diphtheria, tetanus and scarlet fever.

Chapter 4

Body Mechanics and Posture

STANDING POSITION

In correct standing position the head is held erect, back is kept straight as much as possible, chest is put forward, shoulders are kept back, elbows are slightly flexed, wrists are extended, fingers are slightly flexed, abdomen is drawn inward and kept flat, knees are slightly flexed, and feet are pointing ahead and parallel to each other about 3 inches apart. Knowledge of correct.

Standing position is necessary because all other positions are modifications of standing position. When a nurse helps the patient to sit or lie down in bed, she follows the principles of correct standing position and keeps the patient's body in good alignment.

SITTING POSITION

In sitting position, the weight of the body is balanced by ischial tuberosities, the buttocks and the thighs. Elbows are flexed and supported, hips are flexed at right angles to the trunk, knees are flexed at right angles to the thighs, and angles are flexed to right angles to the legs and are flat on floor. Back is held erect and the back and buttocks are supported by the back of the chair.

POSITIONS USED FOR PATIENTS

Dorsal position

Patient is flat on the bed with legs extended and arms at

the sides of the body. This is not a comfortable position, as the curves of the body are not supported.

Dorsal Recumbent Position

This is called back lying position. This is a modification of standing position. The only difference being, the patient is in horizontal position instead of vertical. Patient lies flat on his back with a pillow under his head.

A small pad is placed in the hollow of the back, and the knees are slightly flexed. A soft pillow is arranged under the knees. A footboard is provided to prevent foot drop. Arms are kept at the sides of the body. Most of the patients are nursed in this position.

Lateral Position

Patient lies on his side with spine straight. The knees are flexed; the upper knee is more flexed than the lower one. Pillows may be provided for the head, in between the legs, and to support back and abdomen.

The lower arm is kept above the head and the upper arm is placed on a pillow in front. The arms and legs do not bear the weight of the body. This position is used for general comfort, rest and relaxation. During back care, patient is placed in lateral position. Left lateral position is used for vaginal, perineal and rectal examinations, and the post operative patients are kept in lateral position in order to maintain a clear airway.

Jack Knife Position

Patient lies on his back with his shoulders slightly elevated. The hips and knees are flexed and brought up to the abdomen and chest. This position is useful to perform a lumbar puncture.

Knee chest Position

The patient knees on the bed and then lowers his head, shoulders and chest and rests them on the bed. Head is turned to one side, and kept on a pillow. The thighs are kept vertical. Arms are crossed above the head.

This position is useful for performing vaginal and rectal examinations and for correcting displaced uterus or other organs.

Lithotomy Position

The patient is kept on his back. Head and shoulders rest on a small soft pillow. Knees are flexed well and buttocks are brought over to the edge of the bed. If it is used for a long period, the legs are supported by stirrups, attached to the table. The position is used for examination or operations on rectum and genital organs.

Prone Position

Patient lies flat on his abdomen with head kept on a pillow and turned to one side. Pillows are kept under the waist and under the lower legs. The arms are flexed at the elbow and kept above the head. This position is used when there is bedsore or burns or an injury at the back and as a change of position for patients with fractured spine.

This is a modified left lateral position. The patient lies on the left side. Head, shoulders and chest are turned forward so that her chest rests on the pillow. The right knee is well flexed and rests on the bed in front.

The left knee is slightly flexed and is positioned behind the right knee. This position is useful for performing vaginal examinations and for rest and relaxation. Patient is in a partially sitting position. The back of the bed is elevated to 45 degrees with the aid of a backrest and pillows or by adjustment of the cot. Patient's back, shoulder and head are supported well.

The knees are flexed and supported with a pillow or by cot adjustment. A footrest is provided to prevent foot drop. Patients are not kept in this position for long time, since there is always the danger of thrombus formation. This position is used for patients with dyspnoea (difficulty in breathing), distended abdomen, abdominal surgery, cardio-thoracic disorders and ascites. The position is also useful while passing Ryle's tube and while performing tapping of ascites fluid.

Trendelenburg Position

The patient lies on his back with the foot of the bed elevated on wooden blocks. Patient's head and trunk are lower than the legs.

Reverse Trendelenburg Position

The head and shoulders are at a higher level than the hips, legs and feet. This position is used for reducing intracranial pressure and for other treatment measures.

Moving and Lifting Patient

As nurses, you may be required to move and lift patients. An important point you have to bear in mind while moving patients is that you must observe correct body mechanics for your patients as well as for yourself. While lifting heavy objects, it is wise to stand with your feet while apart and firmly on the floor. The weight should be lifted close to the body. Flex your knees so that your strong muscles of the legs bear the weight of the object.

Purposes

- To perform the task efficiently
- To avoid the patient from unnecessary effort
- The prevent nurses from strain and back injuries
- To promote circulation and muscular tone

Procedures a. Moving upward or downward

Two nurses are required to do this. One nurse places her one hand under the patient's shoulder and the other hand under the lumbar region. The other nurse stands on the other side of the bed and does the same as the first nurse. The patient, if he is able, is asked to flex the knee and push against the matters with heels. Both nurses together bring the patient up.

Moving from one Side of bed to Another

Move pillows towards the side of the bed. Place your one arm under the shoulders and the other under the lumbar region. Move upper part of the body to the side of the bed.

Then keep one arm under the lumbar region and the other under the thighs and move the middle part of the body of the side of the bed. Lastly place one arm under the things and the other under the ankles and move the lower part of the body to the side of the bed. See whether the whole body is straight and in good alignment.

Turning on Side

Before turning move the patient a little away from the centre. If he is to be turned on the left side, you stand at his left. Keep his right arm crossed on the chest and right leg crossed over the left leg. Flex the right knee slightly keep one hand on the patient's right shoulder and the other on his right hip and gently roll him to left lateral position.

Keep the head of the stretcher at right angles to the foot of the bed. Three nurses are needed. All stand on the same side of the stretcher one nurse places her arms under the patient's head and shoulders, another keeps her arms under the hips, the third has her arms under the things and legs. All together life the patient, turn and place him on the bed. The lifters observe body mechanics for themselves. They keep their backs straight, flex their knees and place their one foot forward while transferring the patient.

Chapter 5

Basic Principles of Psychology

PSYCHOLOGY

"Psychology" is a branch of science dealing with knowledge of mind and soul. It plays a vital role in taking care of the patients in nursing. The knowledge of basic principles of psychology is significant in taking care of nurse herself and also in her interaction with the patient. The nurses should understand that the fulfillment of basic needs as given below is imperative in achieving one' s own self actualisation.

Basic Needs

In 1943, five types of human need a hierarchy, from the physiological through safety needs. Love needs. Esteem needs and culminating in a need for self-actualization has been proposed by Maslow, the psychologist.

Physiological Needs

The lowest in the motivation hierarchy includes need for water, oxygen, food, sleep, activity, sex sensory satisfaction etc. A man is never satisfied with all his needs. If one need is satisfied another need will arise and it is human tendency.

Safety Needs

If physiological needs tend to be met consistently and more or less completely the organism expresses the next dwell i.e. the safety needs. We experience safety needs only when there is a threat to its existences. However it is possible to perceive psychological threat, just as one may perceive physical threat. The reaction of such perceptions leads to real conditions of neurosis. Safety needs are decent housing and employment.

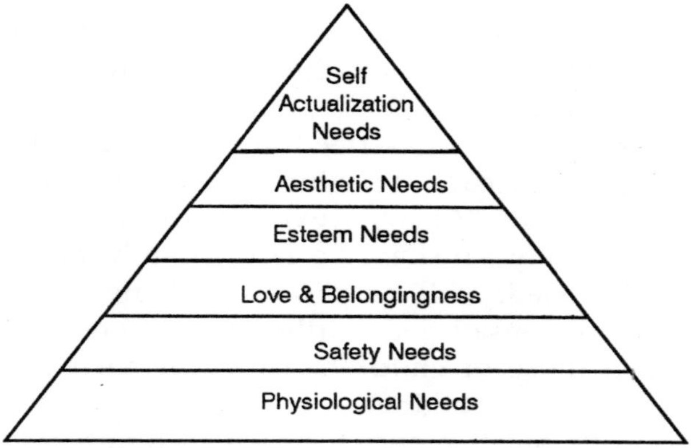
Self
Actualization
Needs
Aesthetic Needs
Esteem Needs
Love & Belongingness
Safety Needs
Physiological Needs

Fig. Maslow' s Hierarchy Theory.

According to Maslow satisfaction of these needs will open the door for expression of the next level of needs.

Love Needs

Love needs encompass all desire for relations with people. They include acceptance by others and achievement of some status within group by which the individual is accepted. Maslow states that lack of satisfaction, in this area is most common source of maladjustment and consequent psychopathological conditions.

Esteem Needs

Each of us has need for self-respect and a need for the respect of others. The former expresses it self as a device for achievement, adequate confidence and the later recognition, attention and rewards from others. When unsatisfied, we feel confident and while when thwarted we feel inferior and helpless. It is an expression of lack of satisfaction of esteem.

Self Actualization Needs

- Self-actualization goes beyond esteem because it

emphasizes becoming whatever one must be. Esteem can be achieved without self-actualization.

- Self-actualization means fulfilling our potential since this never occurs the need can never be satisfied. As the progress is made new possibilities are opened by ones potential and this further striving toward (self) actualization.

  The five needs described above are actually broad categories each of which may contain specific expression. At whatever level, man is never completely satisfied, he is constantly needs, since some needs will be partially satisfied and others partially unsatisfied. Further there are needs of adult than those of children. However such needs are emerging in children.
- So one must interpret, action in terms of relevant needs and make it possible for the child to achieve satisfaction.
- If children find physiological safety, and love needs at least partially satisfied, they will evidence a need for esteem and this may find proper expression through academic achievement. Where need for esteem is not present, that means other lower needs in the hierarchy are being insufficiently met.

  The teacher must first arrange appropriate conditions for their satisfaction, whether in or out of school. Once meeting, esteem needs will be of no problem, though their satisfaction will depend upon self-group variables.

MOTIVATION

"Motivation is an essential condition of Learning process," says Melton. "Motivation represents the antecedent dynamic background for both original behaviour and it' s modifications" says Gates. Motivation is an art if attracting others towards oneself. In many of our activities. Whether personal, social, or national, motivation is present directly or indirectly.

Motivation has become an art of giving incentives to

others for doing something; art of making appeals in order to attract others towards oneself. Needless to add that motivation is useful in nursing profession. In the field of education ends and means are complementary to each other. When we attain something, that something becomes a means for attracting some other thing higher than that.

Thus we are continuously engaged in obtaining our goals and using the same as a means for attaining something higher end. So what was end once becomes a means for another time. Needless to remark, that a number of small ends go to formulate a bigger end. So we are consistently engaged in using an end as a motivation.

In education this type of continuous arousal of motivation is of great importance. There may not be any relationship necessarily between intensity and duration of motivation. If motivation is very intense, the goal is likely to be achieved sooner.

Then if duration will be shorter and if the goal of an intensive motivation is not achieved soon, its duration will be continued till the achievement of the same. Thus an intensive motivation is likely to control the human behaviour for a longer duration. The sphere of motivation depends upon the environment. Our lives will come to an end and all our activities; will be stopped if we do not feel motivated for one thing or another.

Kinds of Motivation

- Natural and artificial,
- Intrinsic and extrinsic.
- Automatic actions and reflexes, habit, instincts, feelings, desire interests, suggestion, imitation are natural motivation.
- To acquire knowledge, to win affection of the person we love, to obtain a post, to acquire confidence of others, to obtain leadership and popularity may be the artificial motivations for an individual.

These may also be regarded as natural because they are found in most of us and many of our activities are guided by them. Artificial motivation have their base in some of our natural motivation, instincts, urges, drives or natural needs. The physical, mental and social development of the individual should be rightly understood for ascertaining what type of artificial motivation will be more appropriate.

The individual will not feel motivated, unless he has a goal to achieve. A model before him will further energize him. Thus he will feel inner striving and this striving will be purposive. So in the presence of a goal, model and purposive striving, a student may be guided to achieve great heights.

The patient must be given a correct knowledge of his progress in order to motivate him further, when he realizes that he is progressing well he puts in greater efforts. Reward is a great motivation.

An individual is naturally desirous of obtaining reward on his successful performance. The fear of punishment goads the individual to follow the right path. Punishment serves as a powerful motivation to follow the right path. Maslow' s proposes a comprehensive theory of need of gratification and growth motivation including fundamental physiological needs.

The main reason why disadvantaged and poor children refuse to be motivated in the classrooms to learn is that their basic bodily needs remain unsatisfied. Under safety needs such as security routine regularity, children do need discipline within their levels of understanding in order to perceive an orderly and organized world.

Often under achievers are the resultant of lack of love and understanding. Esteem needs cover confidence, independence, recognition, attention and appreciation. When the above needs are a satisfied the classroom climate is synergetic and help the individual to actualize his inner potentialities.

Achievement Motivation

Just as Maslow, Murray gives an impressive list of

- Achievement,
- Abasement,
- Aggression,
- Exhibition,

- Defenses,
- Autonomy,
- Dominance,
- Affiliation,
- Occurrences,
- Nurturance and
- Sentience as human motives. Achievement motive is a type of social motive. It appears to be a widely generalized level of aspiration, aiming at excellence in all under taken activities. It involves an exalted self-esteem and self-image and it is a learned motive, acquired in the process of growing up and living in a society.

  In this motivation, the goals set by individuals themselves have energizing properties to motivate behaviour. McClelland, in her study on measurement and application of the achievement motive, symbolically expressed in an arch (need for Achievement) and explained the social origins of achievement motivation and its implications for social progress. McClelland also listed conditions for effective pupil motivation. These are,
- Let pupils understand reasons for developing certain motives,
- Let motives be realistic, link motives with activities and daily life events,
- Commit pupil progress give pupils honest and warm support, encourage self study and make pupil feel that he belongs to some successful group.

Individual Differences

All the living organism differ in size, shape, appearance, speed of reaction and innumerable other aspects of behaviour. We can see that some are healthy and jolly while others are weak and irreparable. Some learn quickly and others slowly. In this way exists there differences.

- These differences between individuals that distinguish or separate them from one another and make one as unique individual in oneself are named as individual differences in psychology.

- Individuals differ in height, weight, colour, structure physically and people differ in intellectual abilities like reasoning and thinking power, power of imagination,creative, expression, concentration etc.

Classifications On the basis, they are usually classified as

- Idiot
- Imbecile
- Moron
- Border like normal bright very superior as genius. T here exist wide differences in motor capacities such as reaction time, speed of action, steadiness, rate of muscular movement, manual dexterity and resistance to fatigue etc. Differences exist
- In achievement and
- In knowledge.

Factors Causing Individual Differences

Here dity and environment are not two independent factors. They operate conjointly to contribute their share but they interact and are inextricably involved in their effect, making each person unique.

The complexity of the environmental influences, prenatal, postnatal, material and social cultural are some of the factors causing individual differences. Bio chemical differences between male and female and sex role expectations incorporated into self-concept very early in life are some of the factors.

Girls display greater social and emotional maturity at each age and boys show greater vitality, independence and initiative. M aintenance of cumulative records for each pupil helps in understanding the specific abilities, needs and interests of each pupil as well as his past history. The fact of individual differences implies that teachers have to meet wide variety of pupil' s needs such as needs of

- Exceptional children,
- Gifted children,

- Slow learners or backward children,
- Children with sensory and motor defects,
- Clumsy children etc. Teachers also face antisocial behaviour of some children in their class. Common behaviour problems are bullying, lying, stealing, destruction of common property and adolescent sexual misbehaviour. Suitable reinforcement of acceptable conduct will generally eliminate such problem behaviours.

Interest William James

The popular psychologist defines "interest as a form of selective awareness of attention that produces meaning out of the mass of one' s experiences" Strong speaks of interests "as likes and labels dislikes as aversions". L et us look upon interests as organic conditions that result in a desire for further stimulator from a particular type of object idea or experiences. Evidences of interests in the form of attention can be observed in the early behaviour of infants.

At first this activity is permanently biological but as perceptions occurs and concepts begin to form, the psychological component becomes more important. The child learns to avoid those activities as unsatisfying and to repeat those that have proved to be worthwhile.

Interest, in fact form an integral aspect of personality and they are not outside personality. Interest largely means the individual' s likes or the individual' s preferences to engage himself in a particular type of work, might have other preferences to another type of work. Interests are also divided into extrinsic or intrinsic interest.

- Extrinsic interest are connected with activities that gives rise to satisfaction or pleasure. Intrinsic interests are those are connected with the activity itself.
- An intrinsic interest centered on the activity itself is more basic or real interest. However the differentiation is not easy.

Sometimes an interest may be intrinsic or sometimes it may be extrinsic. eg Playing volleyball or basketball for sake of playing is an intrinsic interest. The individual desires pleasure from it. Playing the same games to earn a reward or trophy or title is an extrinsic interest. Interests are not like aptitude. They are required by the individual in the course of his development. Some interest may be present at one time and disappear at another. Rarely does an individual' s interest last long. However certain basic interest seems to last long for a lifetime.

An interest is not permanent. it is acquired during the lifetime and it may be modified. At school, we expect the pupils to be interested in reading books, playing games etc. When they grow up and enter working life, some may keep the interest of reading and some may keep the interest of playing. I n terests provide useful information for guidance in education and vocational areas.

There are a number of psychological test to assess or measure interests. The most well known highly sophisticated instrument is Strong ' s vocational interest blank. This is in two forms one for men and another for women.

Strong approached different occupational group, such as physician, surgeon, scientists, university teachers, schoolteachers, lawyers, accountants, engineers etc. More than three hundred occupational group were considered and from each individual be obtained a list of interests and activities the individual liked and disliked. Another tool is used to access interest is Kuder' s preference record. (KRP).

The interests which were rated high by a particular occupational groups were called the interests on mechanical, computational, scientific, persuasive etc. Interpretation of test result is to be made on the basis of appropriate norms provided in the concerned manual.

The highest score indicates the important interest and the lowest least important interest area. The guidance worker with the help of this objective test information obtained from achievement, aptitude, personality and interest can help the pupil to obtain a much better and deeper understanding of his personality. The counsellor also has a better understanding of the counsellee (pupil) and thus can guide him (pupil) better with regard to two major areas of choice namely,

- What courses they may pursue or choose or
- What type of or kind of job, that they may take up. Thus in the areas of educational, vocational guidance tests of interests are of greater value.

ATTITUDE

Attitudes have been defined as ideas with emotional content important beliefs, predispositions, biases and appreciations and as state of readiness or set. Allport has defined attitude "as a mental and neural state of readiness organized through experiences exerting a directive or dynamic influence upon the individual response to all objects with which it is related".

Attitudes have intellectual, biological, social emotional components that are derived from experiences and exercise determining influences upon behaviour.

Variety of patterns of attitudes toward health, life and death of people, new situations, music and art, work, play, government, religion and many more have been influenced by the process through planned and random experiences in creating and shaping attitudes. In this school, family and society play vital roles.

- As the growth and development occurs in the infant a changing array of needs bring new reaction to objects and situations.
- An infant, gains pleasure from being helped and protected where as a child in the early period of walking is likely to and resent and reject the helping hand.
- Development changes of this kind produce tremendous change in the child relationship with objects and situations.
- Despite apparent incongruity, the orderly and sequential development of the total organisms, result in threads of continuity of feeling.
- Ordinarily a satisfying state of affairs over and extended period of time, produces a positive feeling in the child for the object or activity involved.

- As the child's perceptional field expands, generalization of response becomes possible. An infant who has experienced general pleasure at the breast or bottle is likely to anticipate pleasure from eating other foods.
- Continued dissatisfaction and unpleasantness during nursing are likely to create a negative feeling about eating.
- A child attitudes authority figure, is obviously an important element of socialization and determines much of his behaviour in school
- Early experiences involving the child and his parents are responsible for the beginnings of this attitude. A rebellious attitude towards authority figure teachers, Principal, leader etc.
- May spring from a conflict with some one in authority, usually a parent or a parent substitute.
- Another important element in the early development of the attitude toward adult is the satisfaction or dissatisfaction derived from the child' s dependency upon parents particularly the mother figure.
- Any separation from the family and especially from the mother is for a young child a painfull and distressing experience, which is not tolerable before he has acquired the concepts of time and space.
- Such an experience in children under three years of age, usually brings a change in the relationship with adults too.
- Separation over a period of time accompanied by depriving of needs is likely to produce incapacity to achieve close and intimate human relationship.
- The attitude of the child toward the teacher is strongly influenced by the following elements of mother child relationship.
- Satisfying experiences with mother.
- Mother's experience and what she expected of the child.
- Mother's attitudes towards other children in the family.

- The parental attitude of acceptant democratic seems to facilitate growth and development more than the others.
- These children from the home atmosphere of warmth and equality have an accelerated intellectual development are more original, emotionally more secured, less excitable, popular, friendly and non aggressive.

Attitude has four dimensions intensity, direction, extensity and duration. Extensity of an attitude is evidenced by the extent to which it motivates an individual' s behaviour. Limits of interest can be determined by the nature of barriers needed to exhibit a response.

Behaviour motivated by a weak attitude can be the thwarted by the obstacle that seem to have very little actual substance, but an intense attitude is likely to find expression in behaviour despite almost over-whelming obstacles. The dimension of an attitude is observed in behaviour as a force that repels, attracts or fails to motivate the child in any direction as in the case of an I don' t particularly care attitude.

Although behaviour in a given direction frequently indicates directly related attitude, there are numerous occasions when the opposite interpretation is in order. An individual having a negative attitude towards a given group may join them outwardly seeming to have a positive attitude. But by the very subtle means brings about disruption and chaos in the group or divert it from its goal.

Extensity is observed in a broad survey of pattern of attitude within the individual. Some attitudes seem to have broad and pervading influences. The duration of an attitude is another aspect that is important to education. A function of education is the modification of existing negative attitude and creation of new ones that are positive and enduring attitudes may endure only for a short time, because they have not been reinforced by experiences.

Infact new experiences may bring about a complete reverse of the previous attitudes. Attitudes are changed by school experiences. They may be changed by the influence of a particular teacher, another child, peer groups, a single event, curriculum material or a series of extracurricular events. A desirable attitude toward learning will be maintained if

- The thing to be learned is not too far removed from past learning's.
- The learning situations are made physically and intellectually attractive to the learner.
- The knowledge of skill to be acquired is perceived as a need satisfier.
- The concomitant experiences do not appear to be more immediate goal satisfiers.
- Learning in an accompanied by a feeling of achievement reinforced by recognition from others. When these conditions are sustained for all learners' teachers will no longer be troubled by children, who have negative attitudes toward school.

EMOTION

The psychologist Kulpe defines emotion "as a fusion of feeling and organic sensations". The psychologist Hoffding defines it "as a pleasure pain in association with the idea of its cause". According to psychologist Ward, "it is the complete psychosis involving cognition, pleasure-pain and conation". In general emotion "is a complex, not a simple elementary, mental state".

The difference between motives and emotions are as follows: Emotions are usually aroused by external stimuli and that emotional expression is directed toward the stimuli in the environment that arouses it. Motives on the other hand, are more often aroused by internal stimuli and naturally directed towards certain objects in the environment (eg Food, Water). Most motivated behaviour has some affective or emotional accompaniment although we may be too preoccupied in our striving toward the goal. Motivation is focused on the goal directed activity. Emotion is focused on the subjective, affective experiences that accompany behaviour. Emotions are expressed by language, facial expressions and gestures. An emotional state is characterized by

- A more or less pronounced affective tone. Pleasure unpleasure-experienced in connection with some objective or situation.
- A diffuse stimulation of the organic processes, involving pulse, respiration, glandular secretions which is usually called the organic resonance of the emotion but according to theory of the psychologist James Lange, it is identified with emotion itself
- A narrowing and specializing of consciousness, both on the cognitive and on the curative side, the consequence of what we may call emotional disassociation.
- An impulsive force Physiological Changes in Emotions:

All emotional states affect the activities of the salivary glands. The bodily effects of pain hunger fear and rage have all the emotions of characteristically, negative polarity. In such cases the secretion of saliva is diminished or inhibited. There is a fair presumption that emotions of an opposite or positive, polarity will produce the opposite effect but practically no experimental evidence.

The emotional disturbances of a negative polarity (that is disagreeable) involve disturbance of the digestive functions in all its aspects. The flow of saliva is diminished or altogether inhibited, and its chemical composition altered. The flow of gastric juices is similarly diminished or inhibited and altered chemically.

The negative moments then tend to cease. This fact suggested to psychologist Cannon, the possibility that emotional excitement might involve an increased secretion of adenines and that this adenine in the blood might have the effect of prolonging the inhibition of the activity of the digestive glands after the emotional excitement itself had disappeared.

By testing the blood for adenine after a period of time for the quantity of adenine in the blood, it is greatly increased as a result of strong emotion. M ost of the physiological changes that occur during intense emotion, result from activation of the sympathetic division of the autonomic nervous system as it prepares the body for emergency action. The sympathetic system is responsible for the following changes.

- Blood pressure and heart rate increase
- Respiration becomes more rapid
- The pupils of the eye dilate.
- Electrical resistance of the skin decreases.
- Blood sugar level increases to provide more energy
- The blood begins to clot more quickly in the case of wounds
- Mobility of the gastro intestinal tract decreases or stops entirely. Blood is diverted from the stomach and intestines and are sent to the brain and skeletal muscles.
- The hairs on the skin erect causing "Goose pimples. In emotion the sympathetic system also causes epinephrine (adrenaline) and non- epinephrine (non adrenaline). Nerve impulses with sympathetic system, which reach adrenal glands located on the top of the kidneys, trigger the secretion of hormones. They then get into the blood and circulate around the body.

THEORIES OF EMOTION

James Theory

Emotion proposes the following sequences of events in emotional state:

- First we perceive the situation that will produce emotion. Second we react to this emotion. Third we notice our action. The perception of the reaction is the basis of the emotion as we feel and experience it. The major objection to James Lange theory came from Cannon Who pointed out that changes do not seem to differ very much from one emotional state to another.
- The internal organs are relatively intensive structures not well supplied with nerves and internal changes occur too slowly to be a source of emotional feelings.
- Artificially inducing the bodily changes associated

with an emotion injecting a person with adrenaline does not produce the experience of the true emotion.

James Langes Theory

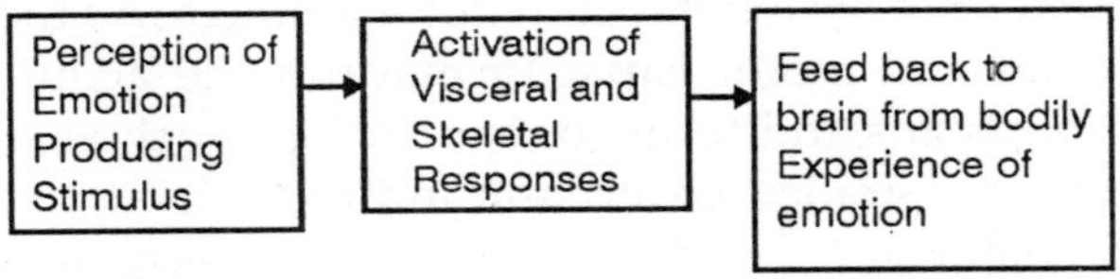

Canon Theory

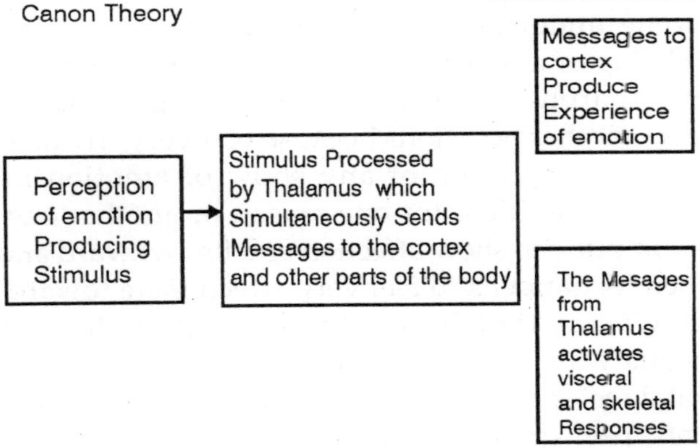

Emotion when sufficiently intense can seriously impair the processes that control organized behaviour. The following diagram illustrate the relationship between the level of emotional arousal and the effectiveness of performance.

Emotional behaviour studies in infancy and early childhood by means of direct observation. Motion pictures and recording of children' s cries indicate that the infants' response to stimuli designated to arouse emotion are very diffuse and lacking in organization.

Emotional shocks and hurts suffered by individuals at an early age can handicap them as long as they live. Children sooner or later acquire the capacity for experiencing negative emotions such as anger, fear and also sorrow or grief to an intense degree. This capacity develops, before the child is mature enough to use language, to formulate his experience in words. F o r a time, the infants' expression of rage is poorly organized. Later his anger becomes more definitely directed at some thing or some body. Changes can likewise be noted in a child' s expression of fear and his reactions to pain. T h e se improv-ements in the young child' s ability to respond in specific ways to situations that arouse him, parallel the development of his mental and motor abilities. As the child ' s intellectual and motor capacity matures, he acquires large variety of means and forms of expressions such as overt and direct to more graded covert and indirect.

The habit of concealing emotion may become especially burdensome under two conditions. If a person may mask intense feeling of anger that occurs when someone hunts his pride very sharply and then still harbouring his anger, may explode on another occasions because of a very trivial affront.

A g ain suppression of any show of emotion may be harmful if an individual for one reason or another has put a lid on any impulse to show affection and its awkward and even rude, when he happens to feel very affectionate toward some one and wishes that he could some how show it in a spontaneous way. The most important factors in a child' s emotional development are the affection that he receives from his parents, peer group and society.

This gives opportunity to develop wholesome affection for his fellow creatures. The more genuine the parents love for the child, the more the child tends to feel free to love other people. More over he is likely to express all his emotions at ease. All physiological healthy nurses are likely to feel some affection for patients in their charge or with whom they have a chance to associate even though the children are not their own. Affection is important for an individual ' s emotional welfare promoting security. The unloved person may suffer in connection with the development of positive attitudes and concepts concerning his own worth.

Adjustment

Adjustment is the process by which living organism maintains a balance between its needs and the circumstances that influence the satisfaction of these needs," says Lawrence F.Shaffer. Accordingly the process of adjustment has two primary main elements:

- One,the needs of the living organism and
- two conditions of the circumstances that influence those needs.

These needs can be biogenic, originating in society, personal or communal, On the other hand, the circumstances influencing these needs also can either be inside the individual or outside him. Factors with in the individual that influence these needs are his physical and mental states capacity, attitudes, interests etc. For example most weakly constituted individuals cannot fulfill their own psychological motives and thus their needs are definitely affected by their lack of strength factors.

Arising within the environment are usually geographic conditions, social conditions, political and cultural influences. These conditions and circumstances can help as well as deter the fulfillment of the individual' s requirements. In this manner, the nature of influences upon the person' s needs is of two kinds, where one is favorable and the other unfavorable. Positive or favorable influences help in the fulfillment of needs while unfavorable influences hinder their satisfactions. These elements in adjustment are

- Motive
- Thwarting conditions
- Varied Responses.

Motive

The very process of adjustment in the living being is set in motion by the presence of motive within him, or needs or requirement from outside. When the environment does not present any features that tend to become obstacles in the fulfillment of these needs, then the adjustment is natural, facile and effortless and no problem result. But if circumstances create obstacles in the path of such fulfillment, then the process of adjustment progresses further.

Varied Responses

Once the fulfillment of a need has been obstructed, the individual indulges in various actions, which are reaction to the obstacle. Such a reaction can be normal just as much as it can be abnormal. Solution: As a result of these reaction and responses, the individual achieves a degree of adjustment with the circumstances. The problem of adjustment in thereby solved. An Exsmple A student is actuated by a strong desire to stand in his class and to do so by scoring very well. He works extremely hard but fails to achieve his objective because he has not the necessary mental equipment i.e. lack of the requisite intelligence.

This forms an obstacle to the satisfactory of this motive and hence as a result the student condescends to lower his aim some what by aiming at securing a second division. In order to accommodate this change of objective, the student changes the mode of study. A change of response suitable modification of the objective and the objective prevails. Such a process of adjustment in an universal phenomenon and is seen to be at every level of life, at various times and under varied conditions.

Motives and Adjustment

The process of adjustment can be set in motion by any motive. Physical needs do not have much importance for on the one hand they are easily satisfied. On the other, in the event of their dissatisfaction, life itself ceases in the organism, thus obviating all further adjustment activity.

Hence social motives and requirements have greater importance for the adjustment process. Social motives are developed within a cultural environment. Individuals' of different cultures have different motives and different cultures do not generate identical motives. Once they have been excited then can only have strong motives satisfied. Inability to satisfy them only leads to further dissatisfaction and this tension is not ended till the objectives have been attained.

Thwarting in Adjustment

Many of the form that thwarting can take and is known to take one form in frustration. For an example if a person fails to catch a train and reach his destination because his wristwatch was not functioning properly, then he has to face frustration that arises out of the environment. Another form is conflict. A state of conflict is precipitated when the individual is actuated by more than one motive arising simultaneously.

Among the classical examples of state of conflict and indecision is the state of the mind of Arjuna as described in the Geeta, when he was divided between war and peace. The state of conflict and tension will continue till the individual decides upon one particular motive. And if the conflict continues the, individual shows signs of mental illness and other abnormalities of behaviour and conduct. Frustration and conflict are closely related.

If the child' s normal expression of aggression and violence restricted from some frustration it becomes repression and gives rise to feelings of fear and insecurity. The individual with an adjustment and organized personality maintains a balance and practical outlook on life. Failures and frustrations do not disturb him and he persists in looking calm and master of the situation. His emotions, needs thinking and other mental activities are adequately balanced and systematized.

On the other hand, the personality of a mal adequate person is non-integrated. Absence of adjustment results in the increase of tension, while its presence helps in reducing tension. Adjustment can be evaluated by the assessment of intensity of tension existing in mind. The methods of adjustment are as follows

Constructive Adjustment

The main feature in this is that it offers a quality of facing the situation rather than running away from and of making efforts that solve the problem instead of merely postponing. EG: When a trader is faced with some problem of his trade, he resorts to exercise economy in expenditure or some other constructive adjustment to solve that problem.

Substitute Adjustment

A large number of individuals have recourse to substitute

adjustments while facing difficult situations. EG: Failure leads to school dropouts. The students start avoiding school since he is defamed and then this obstructs his social motives. Running away ends tension created through this obstruction. Thus for these reasons these reactions to difficult situations are called substitute reactions.

Defense Mechanisms

Another mode of reacting to difficulties is that of mental mechanism or defense oriented reactions to stress aims chiefly at protecting the self from hurt and disorganizations.

Ego Defense Mechanisms

It may be emphasized that the above defense mechanism are, learned. They are designed to deal with inner hurt, anxiety and self-devaluation. They operate on relatively automatic and habitual levels and they typically involve some measure of self-deception and reality distortion. The excess use of the above defense mechanism will lead to mental illness.

PERSONALITY

The word personality has been derived from the Latin word ' Persona' which was the mask which Greek actor work while acting. This however is not the meaning taken in the modern word personality. This personality is not fixed state but a dynamic totality, which is continuously changing due to interaction with the environment.

Personality is known by the conduct, behaviour, activities, and movements. It is the way of responding to the environment. The way in which the individual adjusts with the external environment is personality.

Definition of Personality

In the words of Munn, it is the characteristic integration of an individual' s structure, modes of behaviour, interests, attitudes, capacities, abilities and attitudes. Behaviour requires integration. In the words of Gordon All port, "personality is the dynamic organization within the individual of those psychophysical systems, that determine his unique adjustment to his environment". The personality is the organization of the internal and external activities. It is not a collection of traits but a particular organization of them. Personality is the total quality of behaviour,attitudes, interests, capacities, aptitudes and behaviour patterns, which are manifested in his relation with the environment. An integrated personality leads to organized character.

Disintegrated personality leads to disorganized character. Abnormalities in personality hamper, the organization of character. In mental patient, both character and personality are in disorder. The basic sources of personality development are heredity and environment. However as a persons genetic inheritance interacts with and is shaped by environmental factors, there emerges a self structure that becomes an important influence in shaping further development and behaviour.

Trait and Type Approaches of Personality

The trait approaches to personality attempts to list a number of basic personality traits and the personality of an individual can be described by its position on a scale of units in each of these traits. A trait is an enduring and consistent characteristic of a person that is observed in a wide variety of situations. The traits are intelligence, emotional sensitivity ascendance, submission, irritable, warm etc. In fact All port and Odbert have listed 17,953 words in English, which are adjectives standing for personality traits. He distinguished between surface traits and source traits.

CATTELL

Cattell has startrd 16 personality factors as primary or source traits. Allport distinguished cardinal traits (basic) central traits, and secondary traits. Some of the traits mentioned by are

Norman listed 5 terms extroversion, agreeableness, conscientiousness, emotional stability and culture. H.J.Evsenck speaks of three basic categories of personality.

Genial	⟷	Hostile
Intelligence	⟷	Stupid
Emotionally	⟷	Stable Chargeable,
Dominant	⟷	Submissive,
Cheerful	⟷	Unhappy,
Co-Operation	⟷	Reserved,
Hypersensitive	⟷	Phlegmatic,
Friendly	⟷	Suspicious etc

- *Extroversion:* Introversion,
- *Neuroticism:* Stability
- *Psychotism normality:* This has been ultimately reduced to stable unstable and introversion extroversion.
- Extroverts are described as outgoing, uninhibited fond of activities, which bring them into contact with other people. Introverts have the opposite traits.
- Neurotism stability in Evsenchk' s model ranges from stability to high anxiety. In situations of worry, panicking, stress and over emotionality a high level activity could affect performance adversely in academic work of pupils, resulting in learning disabilities. The type approach It is older than the trait approach, which depends upon modem statistical procedures.

Hippocrates and Galen have associated personalities with certain kinds of body fluids called humors. Galen has spoken of four kinds of human temperaments

- Choleric,
- Melancholic,
- Phlegmatic and
- Sanguine. Krrlchmer refers to following types of human personality based on bodily fluid. These are
- Aesthenic (thin, long) who are shy and sensitive, withdrawn,
- Pyknic (short fat) who are jovial outgoing with fluctuating moods.

- Athletic (strong and sturdy). The athletic and asthenic type of body build, go with what is known as schizothyme personality and the pyknic body goes with cyclothymic' s personality. The former is basically interested in him only and the latter extroverted. Sheldon speaks of three types of body build
- Endomorphic (round fat and muscular)
- Mesomorphy (hard and muscular) and
- Ectomorphy (delicate and lean).
- Endomorpic individuals have the type of personality called viscerotonia - which implies love of leisure, desire for food and sleep.
- Mesomorphs have somatotomic personalities, who exhibit persistence in behaviour desire for adventure, courage and involvement in actions.
- Ectomorphs have cerebrotonia which implies disciplined behaviour, ready response to stimulation, lack of interest in social interaction, hypersensitivity to pain etc. The most popular theory of Jungs, Extroversion and introversion also is not universally accepted since he himself saves that most persons appear to be a typical ambiverts.

Psychological Theories of Personality

Personality theories are grouped under three major heads (a) Psychodynamic theories (Frend and Jung b) Social learning theories (of Dollard and Miller) (c) Phenomenological theories (Rogers and Maslow)

Psychodynamic Theories of Personality

Psychoanalytic theories of personality are referred to as psychodynamic theory. This theory attempts to understand personality in terms of mental functions may be rational. Irrational, conscious or unconscious.

Freud' s theory of psychoanalysis emphasizes man as dynamic system of energies and the main storehouse of such energies is unconscious. The contents of the unconscious invariably exhibit conflicts. To Freud, the structure of an individual' s Personality consists of 3 separate agencies;

- Id is the inborn reservoirs of primitive psychic energy called libido, unconscious demanding immediate satisfaction on the basis of pleasure principle regardless of external which ego and superego develops and it consists of energy thing that is inherited.
- All the energy of human behaviour is provided by two inborn id instincts namely sex and aggression, which he spoke of Eros-life instincts and thantoes, death instincts.
- Ego embodies a rational cognitive capacity that demands of super ego.
- Id seeks pleasure ego test reality and super ego strives for perfection. From Anxiety, defense mechanism or unconscious attempts to reduce anxiety by denying or destroying reality. The technique of Eric Berne' s transactional refers to wholesome transaction from childhood to adulthood. Freud also emphasizes the early experiences in personality development. He speaks of psychosexual development of the individual.
- The oral stage, during infancy and
- The anal stage between the age 2 and 3,
- The phallic stage 3 to 5,
- From 5 up to early adolescence the stage of Oedipuscomplex/electracomplex. Then from 5 up to early adolescence sexual force are subordinated which marks the latency, period and finally the genital stage of heterosexuality.
- Psychosexual maturity is reached by an individual as the end result of successful passage through the full sequence of stages.

Carl Jung differs from Preud in taking a more positive and optimistic attitude towards human nature believing that people not only try to gratify their instincts but also try to develop their potential. Jung agreeing with Freudian view of unconsciousness, which represents the accumulated experiences, and culture of the human species throughout its evolutionary development from primitive times. Alfred Adler' s personality theory stress the uniqueness of one' s personality looks upon aggression is more significant than sex as a motive of behaviour.

He points to the innate striving for superiority. To Erikson, personality is the resultant from interaction between the needs of a person and the demands of a society at a particular stage of development. He refers to eight psychosocial stages of development. A particular type of crisis characterizes each stage. Ego identify crisis during adolescence and now an individual resolves such crises determines personality characteristics.

H.S.Sviiilan has stressed the interpersonal nature of personality and has laid on the acquisition of language as a means of normal personality development. Social learning theories of personality. These theories say that consistency of behaviour, results not only from rigid personality traits but also from other factors like environmental stability. Skinner and hull' s learning theories are based on the above factors. Dollard and Miller pointed fear, as an important factor in personality development as it acts as a powerful motive or drive in the promotion of learning.

The ' role' theory of G.H.Mead speaks of different roles one plays in life (a son, pupil, leader, friend etc) and gradually internalizes the associated traits to form his personality. A person' s behaviour depends upon the specific nature of the situation, how the situation is appraised by him as well as past reinforcement of behaviour in similar situations.

BEHVOIRISTS THEORIES OF PERSONALITY

Behavoists is such a skinner emphasize that conditioning alone is not adequate to explain human character and personality.

Phenomenological Theories of Personality

This includes humanistic conceptions of personality.

These theories emphasize the existence of positive growth promoting forces in personality beyond more conflict resolution or tension reduction and also stresses present rather than past experiences. Maslow' s theory emphasizes inherent potentialities to seek self-actualization.

Maslow & CarlRoger both dealt on humanistic and psychoanalytic theories on growth and self actualisation. Roger' s client centered on non-directive counselling is popular. The most important concept is self. An individual with a strong positive self-concept seek growth and have pleasant productive relation with others. G.Kelly' s cognitive theory of personality consists of personal constructs that is the ways a person has of evaluating himself and his circumstances.

Assessment of personality

The oldest methods of measuring personality are

- Astrology,
- Palmistry,
- Phrenology etc. More scientific techniques have been evolved to measure personality, which is very helpful in the field of education, employment and medicine. In the field of education, to provide suitable courses, in the field of employment to select suitable person as per the requirements of a job and in the field of medicine to diagnose the mental diseases of patients for giving proper treatments. Some of them are
- Observation,
- Case Study,
- Rating Scale,
- Questionnaire,
- Interview,
- Projective techniques
- *Observation:* There are two types of observation
- Participant
- Non-participant To make observation more effective the observation can make use of tape recorders. Cameras and binoculars. Carefully intelligent and scientific observation is needed in observation method.

- Case study: P.V.Young says case study is a method of exploring and analyzing the life of a social unit be that a person, a family an institution cultural group or even entire community.

Characteristics of Good Case Study

- Adequacy
- Validity
- Continuity
- Confidentiality
- Feed back

Steps in Case Study

- Initial status
- Collection of exploratory data
- Diognosis of causal factors
- Looking forward to remedial development.
- Follow up process.

Rating Scale

- Rating scale is used to quantify an observation. In this method a number of questions are asked to enable a person to rate himself or to enable others to do so. Teacher can use rating scales to categorize their students on a specific trait. Example for self-rating

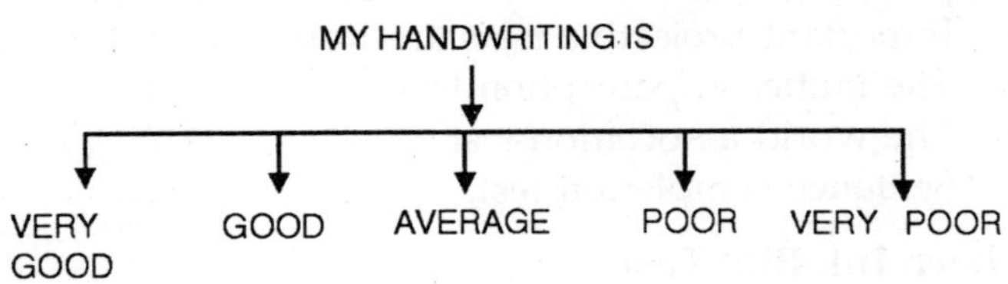

- In spite of faulty logic error, central tendency error and generosity error, it is used for rating students well in scholarship and the quality or leadership sincerity punctuality and honesty.

Questionnaire

It is most popular method useful in collecting quantitative

and qualitative information. A questionnaire should collect information which is normally not available from others sources. It should be arranged in categories to ensure accurate responses.

It should provide complete and clear direction, simplicity, familiarity, singularity, should be used. T he questionnaire should avoid questions of ambiguity, variety it should not be too lengthy. It should be printed Both the methods of mailing and personal contact of administering the questionnaire have their own advantages and disadvantages.

Interview

I n terview is a technique of getting information directly from the subject. It is subjective in nature hence its findings should be supplemented with other methods.

Projective Techniques

P rojective techniques are used to study the unconscious aspect of behaviour, it permits or encourages wide variety of responses and it is highly multidimensional. Drever defines, a projective technique is interpretations of situations and events by reading into them their own experiences and feelings. A Projective techniques is used for

- Clinical settings for digonostic use with the mental patients
- Important projective tests are Rorschach ink blot test
- The maticc apperception test
- The world association test
- Sentence completion test.

Rorschach Ink Blot Test

Rorschach ink blot test: is made up of ten ink blot patterns. 5 are in black and white, two are black and red and 3 are multicolored.

While administering the test encouragements is given when there is no response from the individual. All the responses are taken down verbatim. It does not impose time limits. The scoring categories are named as

- Location
- Content
- Timing
- Determinants
- Originality. Thematic Apperception test developed Murray and Morgan consists of 30 pictures which portray human beings in a variety of actual life situations and 1 black card 10 for male, 10 for female and 10 for both.

  The maximum number of pictures used with any subject is 20. The system of scoring taken into account of the following.
- Hero of the story
- Needs and conflicts of the hero
- Theme of story: the global view should be based upon, the responses of all the 20 pictures shown to the subject and the experiences of the examiner.

Word Assiciation Test

It is of two types:

- Controlled
- Uncontrolled In controlled word association, the subject is given the word and is asked to give the antonym or synonym. In uncontrolled word association, the subject is given a word and asked to reply and the first word that comes to his mind spontaneously is taken into account. The interpretation of the tests depends on two factors (i.e.) the response word and reaction time. Inability to make any response or mere repetition of the stimulus word indicates one's emotional blocking.

Sentence Completion Tests Consists

Sentence completion tests consists of a list of incomplete sentences, generally open at the end and requires completion by the subject who is asked to go through the list and answer as quickly as possible.

On the basis of these responses, the psychologist' s records observation, which indicate unhealthy or conflicting, healthy or positive attitude etc. Stimulus in the form of the following words may be represented.

- I wish to become---------
- My Mother----------
- My Teacher-----------

The above-mentioned incomplete sentences can be completed in many ways. From these answers, we can assess the personality of an individual.

Chapter 6

Hygiene-Patient and Environment

Patient and his environment including the bed comprises of patients unit, which needs to be maintained facilitating hygienic environment helping the cure process.

The word hygiene refers to "the science of health and its maintenance, the prevention of disease, and sanitary practices".

PERSONAL HYGIENE

Personal Hygiene is the activity of self-care, including bathing and grooming. Care of the skin, hair, nails, mouth, teeth, eyes, ears, nasal cavities, and perineal and genital areas.

Factors Influencing Personal Hygiene Practices

- *Development level*: Children learn most of their hygiene practices at home and in their personal environment. They modify their behaviour with other family members.

  Many of these behaviours stick with them throughout life. The advancing age, hormonal levels and changes in the integumentary system often require hygienic practices.
- *Cultural background*: Norms related to hygiene practices differ from culture to culture. For example, North American culture places a high value on personal cleanliness and people have a habit of bathing daily where as people from other culture mayor may not consider bathing as a daily practice.
- *Socio Economic Status*: Financial status often affects a person' s ability to purchase hygiene products.

- *Religion:* Some religions observe specific rules related to personal hygiene.
- *Health status:* Persons who are ill are often unable to attend to personal hygienic activities, either because they have a low energy supply or a specific physical deficit.

Patient and his Bed Bed Making

Bed making is an art. Skillful bed making contributes materially to the patient' s comfort. Clean and comfortable bed includes the patient' s unit in the hospital.

Purpose

- To provide clean and comfortable bed to the patient
- To observe and prevent patient' s complications
- To save time, effort and material
- To provide a neat appearance of the ward/ unit
- To adapt the needs of the patient

Equipments

Open (Simple) Bed

- Bed
- Duster
- Chair and stool
- Protective sheet
- Bed linen, i.e. mattress, mattress cover, bottom sheet one, draw sheet one, pillow, pillow cover, top sheet one, one or more blankets with blanket covers or one counterpane or bedspread in winter.

Closed (Unoccupied) Bed

Supplies as above Occupied Bed

- Chair
- Duster
- Cover sheet
- Fresh linen as necessary.

Admission Bed

- Supplies as in open bed

Post-operative Bed

- Supplies as in open bed except pillow.
- Exfra supplies
  - A tray containing, bowl of gauze pieces, forceps, mouth guard or tongue forceps, airway, small towel, small protective sheet and anaesthetic sheet and towel.
  - Kidney tray, paper bag, safety pins.
  - Shock blocks, intravenous stand.
  - Sterile drainage bag with rubber tubing and a glass connection if patient comes with urinary catheter.
  - 2-3 hot water bottles with covers or other means of warming the bed in winter.

Fracture Bed

- Supplies as in open bed.
- Extra supplies, i.e. fracture boards, bed cradle, sand bags, cover sheet, hot water bottles with covers, if required.

Plaster Bed

- Supplies as in fracture bed.
- Extra supplies, i.e., protective sheet and draw sheet, sand bags and draw sheet heat cradle or electric heater or hot water bottles with covers if required.

Amputation or Stump Bed

- Supplies as in plaster bed.
- Extra supplies i.e. extra set of top clothes, a pillow covered with protective cover and cotton cover, tourniquet and shock blocks.

Cardiac Bed

- Supplies as in open bed.
- Extra supplies, i.e., back rest, pillows 4-5, foot rest board, cardiac table.

Blanket (Rheumatism or Renal) Bed

- Supplies as open bed
- Extra supplies
  - Long protective sheet one, bath sheets two, electric blanket or ordinary woolen blankets-two or more.
  - Bed cradle or hot water bottles with covers.
  - Pillows or sand bags.

GUIDELINES

- The beds are of two types, ordinary and special beds.
  Ordinary Bed
  - Open (simple) bed: This is prepared for an ambulatory patient.
- Indication
  - Provide a clean smooth comfortable bed to the patient.
  - Closed (unoccupied) bed: This is an empty bed in which the top covers are arranged in such a way that all linen beneath the counterpane or bedspread is fully protected from dust and dirt until the admission of new patient. On arrival of the patient, this bed is converted into open bed.
- Indication
  - Keep the bed ready for receiving the new patient.
  - Occupied bed: This bed is prepared for bed-ridden patient, lying in the bed.
- Indication
  - Provide a clean and comfortable bed with the least disturbance of the patient in it.

Special Beds

  - Admission bed This is prepared for the newly admitted patient.
- Indications
  - Provide minimum disturbance to the patient during admission bath and physical examination.
  - Protect bed linen during admission bath and leave a fresh bed immediately ready for the use.

- Post-operative bed. This is prepared for the patient who has undergone surgery.

- Indications
  - Protect bed linen from vomiting, bleeding, drainage and discharges.
  - Provide warmth and comfort to the patient to prevent shock.
  - Fracture bed This is a hard firm bed designed for the patient with fracture particularly of spine, pelvis or femur.
- Indications
  - Aid in immobilizing the fracture.
  - Prevent unnecessary pain.
  - Provide warmth and comfort to the patient.
  - Prevent undue sagging of the mattress.
  - Plaster bed This is a hard bed designed for the patient with plaster.
- Indications
  - Aid in immobilizing the part until the plaster dries.
  - Aid in drying the plaster in correct position and shape.
  - Provide warmth to dry the plaster and keep the patient comfortable.
  - Amputation or stump bed: In this type of bed the top bed clothes are divided or split. This is known as amputation or stump bed when it is used for the patient with amputation of legs.
- Indications
  - Avoid disturbance to the patient during constant observation, repeated applications or treatments are necessary for abdomen or lower limbs. ii Take the weight of the clothes off the side of the amputated limb or stump. iii Keep the stump in good position. iv Watch stump for hemorrhage constantly and apply a tourniquet instantly if necessary.
  - Cardiac bed This is prepared for a patient with heart disease.

- Indications
  - Relieve dyspnoea.
  - Assist in recovery of the patient.
  - Provide comfort to the patient.
  - Prevent complications.
  - Rheumatism or renal bed: This is prepared to provide extra warmth to the patient.
- Indications
  - Provide extra warmth to the body incase of general debility and shock. ii Provide comfort to the aching joints in patients with acute rheumatism.
  - Improve perspiration for excretion of waste products incase of nephritis.
- Burns bed This is prepared for a patient with burns.
- Indications
  - Prevent infection to the burnt area.
  - Help in healing of the burnt area.
  - Provide comfort to the patient.
  - Prevent the patient from sticking to the sheet as a result of exudates oozing from the burnt area.
- The beds must be versatile and adaptable to different needs of the patients with following arrangements.
  - Siderails These are used to
- Prevent the patient from falling out of bed.
- Protect the restless patient.
- Provide the patient support to grasp and hold when moving about.
  - Handcranks These are located at the foot of bed and used to:
- Adjust the height of bed.
- Raise or lower the head, foot or knee sections in order to maintain various bed positions for treatment or comfort.
  - Special attachments The attachments of various poles, frames and equipment for traction are used to modify the beds to meet various needs of the patient for treatment and comfort.

- Collect all the supplies which are likely to be required, place on the stool or bedside table.
- Use a damp duster for enamel painted iron bed and dry one for the varnished bed. Dust mattress and sheets with dry duster and furniture with damp duster.
- When stripping the bed, strip in the following manner:
  - Loosen the bedding all around starting from the head end and proceed to the foot end. Lift the mattress while loosening it.
  - Pick up gently, do not pull with force, shake gently and fold the clean linen which can be used again.
- Fold the counterpane or bed spread twice bringing the top end to the bottom end and then pick up from the centre.
- Fold the other top clothes the same manner.
- Fold the draw sheet in two.
- Roll the protective sheet to prevent creases on it.
- Fold the other bottom clothes as top clothes.
- Place the folded clean linen which can be used again, over the back of the chair and those, which cannot be used, again should be thrown in the dirty linen receptacle. Never throw the soiled linen on the floor to prevent spread of microorganisms.
- Turn the mattress top to bottom or from side to side.
- Turn the pillow.
- Air the cotton mattress and pillow to keep them fresh and soft. Most of the dunlop mattresses are smooth on one side only.
- When the patient is incontinent or has profuse drainage, use protective sheet under the patient.
- Two nurses should work together to make the bed for helpless patient opposite to one another or at each side of the bed.
- Modify the bed according to the weather, needs and habits of the patient.

- When tucking the bed linen under the mattress, pull the sheets with both hands and the palms face down in order to protect your knuckles from bed springs. 10. Never discard woolen blankets in the receptacle along with the soiled clothes. If soiled, treat them separately.
- Make the bed firm, smooth and free of wrinkles.
- After completing the bed making, arrange the locker, bed and bedside furniture properly.
- When making an occupied bed, make every effort to minimize the discomfort to the patient.
- When the patient is in traction, the bed is made without disturbing the traction weights.
- Inspect bed and bedding for vermin and treat accordingly, if present.
- Do not let your uniform touch the bed and bed linen.
- Observe patient' s physical condition to assess patient' s ability for self care.
- Develop relationship (nurse-patient) with the patient.
- The following are the principles of bed making which need to be kept in mind while making bed.
  - Barrier nursing to prevent cross infection.
  - Clean and comfortable bed to ensure rest and sleep and prevent complications.
  - Appropriate body mechanics to maintain body alignment and prevent fatigue.
  - Organised functioning to save time, effort and material.
- Keep in mind the nursing principles while making bed.

Nursing Activity

- Collect and take the supplies to the bed side.
- Place the supplies on the stools.
- Tidy the shelves and move the locker a little away.
- Explain the patient that you are going to make his or her bed.
- Maintain patient' s privacy by using screen.

- Wash your hands.
- Make the bed as mentioned below accordingly

Open Bed

- Assist the patient out of bed as necessary and offer chair to sit.
- Remove any equipment attached to the bed linen.
- Adjust the bed in flat position to a comfortable height to prevent straining your back.
- Strip the bed clothes, fold them one by one and place on the back of a chair, incase to be reused. Remove the mattress cover and bed cover, fold and keep them also
- Dust the bed with damp duster and mattress with dry duster. Turn the mattress
- Spread the bed cover on the bedsprings to protect the under surface of the mattress. Put on the mattress cover, if it is loose the excess can be tucked under the mattress. Pull the mattress to the top.
- Place the bottom sheet at the foot of bed, seam side down with the lower hem even with the edge of the mattress and the centerfold on the centre of the bed. Then, unfold the upper layer onto the head of bed.
- Tuck in excess sheet at the head of the bed
- Miter the corner as below at the head end of bed, making smooth and neat corner.

- Pick up the side edge of the sheet, so that the sheet forms a triangle with the head of bed and the side edge perpendicular to the bed.
- Hold the sheet against the side of mattress using the palm of your hand and tuck the excess sheet under the mattress.
- Drop the sheet from your top hand to the side of mattress.

- Miter the corner as above at the foot end of bed.

- Tuck the sheet under the mattress from head to foot of bed on one side.
- Place a protective sheet and drawsheet in the middle of the bed with the centerfold on the centre of bed and unfold. Then tuck in on one side.
- Place the top sheet at the head of bed, seam side up with the top hem even with the head of mattress and the centerfold on the centre of bed, then unfold the upper layer on to the foot of the bed.
- In winter, placed the blanket and bedspread over the top sheet as under.

• Place the blanket over the top sheet, at the head of bed, about 6-8 inches below the top sheet with the centerfold of the blanket on the centre of bed. Unfold the blanket on the centre of bed. Then unfold the upper layer onto the foot of the bed.

• Place the bedspread on the blanket
  - Make a vertical or horizontal toe pleat as under while tucking the top bedclothes at the foot of the bed.

• Vertical pleat-Fold a six inches pleat lengthwise in the top clothes from the centre to the foot end, at the centre of mattress.

• Horizontal pleat-Fold a two inches pleat across the top clothes at the centre of foot of the mattress.
  - Tuck in the excess sheet, blanket and bedspread together at the foot of the bed.
  - Miter the corner of top clothes at the foot of bed as in step i allowing the top linen to hang over the side of the bed. r. Repeat the procedure on the opposite side, if you do not have other nurse to help you on the other side. Pull the linen tight and smooth out any wrinkles.
  - Fold back the top sheet at the head of the bed to the shoulder height. If blanket and bedspread are used, fold back the top sheet over the edge of

  - blanket and bedspread.
  - Put a clean pillow cover on pillow and place the pillow at the centre of the head of bed, with open end of the cover away from the door of the room.
  - Fanfold the top clothes toward the foot of the bed or pie fold them as under for easy entering.
- Fanfold Fold the half of the top clothes toward the foot of the bed which is further folded into 2-3 accordianpl-eats so that the top clothes are at the foot end of the bed.
- Pie fold Place one finger at the centre of the top clothes facing the head of bed. Lift the edge of the top clothes and fold it back toward the centre of the bed, making a triangle.

Closed Bed

  - The procedure is the same as in open bed except for the bedspread.
- Place the bedspread, keeping seam side down with its centerfold on the centre of the bed.
- Unfold the spread on to the head side of bed, adjust the top edge of spread even with the edge of mattress, tuck in and miter the corners.
- Unfold the spread onto the foot side of bed, tuck in and miter the corners.
  - Follow the steps as mentioned above to convert this bed into an open bed, on the arrival of the new patient.

Occupied Bed

  - Lower the siderails. Strip the bed and replace the top clothes by a cover sheet (top sheet can be used, incase it is not soiled).
  - Fold top clothes one by one to remove and place on the back of the chair in case to be reused.
- Bedspread Fold it in half, top edge to bottom edge or longitudinally with side edge to side edge. Grasp the centre and fold in half, then in half one more time.
- Blanket Fold it as above.

- Top sheet Fold it as above.
  - Move the patient and mattress well up in the bed.
  - Turn the patient towards you.
  - Fold or roll the unclean draw sheet, protective sheet, bottom sheet, one by one as close to the patient' s back as possible, soiled side inward, on the far side of the bed.
  - Dust the mattress thoroughly. Place the clean bottom sheet, protective sheet, draw sheet on the far side and fold or roll the excess bottom clothes one by one close to the patient.
  - Raise the far side rail. Turn the patient away from you. Patient may hold the far side rail for support.
  - Roll the unclean bottom clothes on the near side towards you and remove.
  - Dust the mattress and unroll the clean bottom clothes towards you.
  - Straighten the bottom clothes tight and smooth out wrinkles, tuck these one by one firmly under the mattress and miter the corners.
  - Replace the cover sheet by top clothes.
  - Repeat the steps as mentioned in preparing the open bed. N.B: If the patient cannot be turned, the bottom clothes are changed from head to foot. The bed linen is changed after giving bath to the patient.

Admission Bed

- Prepare the bed as an open bed.
- Fanfold the top clothes neatly to the foot end ofbed.
- Cover the bed with long protective sheet and two bath sheets. Turn down the top bath sheet to the shoulder height and fanfold it lengthwise towards the locker. Place hot water bottles between the blankets to warm the bed in winter.
- Adjust the height of bed to the level of stretcher,

if necessary. N.B: After giving bath, turn the patient towards you, roll the bath sheet and protective sheet and keep close to the patient' s back. Turn the patient to the other side, remove bath sheet and protective sheet and cover the patient with top clothes.

Surgical Bed

- Prepare the bottom of the bed as in open bed.
- Place top clothes on the bed but do not tuck in. Fold them using any one of the following methods.
  - Fold the sides to the middle, then top and bottom to the middle, thus making a packet in the centre of the bed which can be easily moved for the reception of the patient. Place this packet over the hot water bottles in winter.
  - Turn down the top clothes to the shoulder height and then fanfold toward the locker, having the other side clear for receiving the patient. Place hot water bottles in the middle of the bed under the fanfolded top clothes in winter.
- Instead of pillow, place a small protective sheet and a towel on the head end of bed.
- Keep the tray (mentioned in supplies) on the locker or table nearby and shock blocks on floor near the foot end of the bed ready incase of necessity.
- Adjust the height of the bed to the level of the stretcher. N.B: When the patient is received in bed, place kidney tray on the bed near the mouth and pin up the paper bag with the bottom sheet on the side.

Fracture Bed

- Place the fracture board directly over the bedsprings.
- Make the bed as in open bed and spread cover

sheet between the bottom and top clothes. Place hot water bottles in between, to warm the bed in winter.

- Place the sand bags to support the part in order to maintain the position.
- When the patient is received in bed, place the bed cradle over the fractured part between the cover sheet and top clothes to take off the weight of the clothes.

Plaster Bed

Prepare the bed as fracture bed.

- Put on protective sheet and draw sheet where the plaster parts are to be placed to protect the bed linen.
  - Keep the sand bags covered with draw sheet to support the part so that the plaster dries in correct position and shape.
  - When the patient is received in the bed, keep bed cradle over the plastered part between the cover sheet and top clothes to take the weight of the clothes off the plastered part.
  - If possible, the patient may be exposed to the sun rays and if not, then use heat cradle or electric heater. If this is also not possible or available, use hot water bottles to dry the plaster. N.B: Any part of the patient, not covered by the plaster, must be kept warm with a blanket and if the feet are exposed, they may be covered with warm woolen socks.

Divided Bed

- Prepare the bottom of bed as in plaster bed.
- Arrange two sets of top clothes in such a fashion that they are divided in the middle so that the gap will come where it is required.
- Place a pillow covered with protective cover and cotton cover under the stump for support. Sand bags covered in a draw sheet are also placed on the sides

to support the limb in order to keep the stump in good position.

- Tie the tourniquet to the bed loosely to apply instantly when hemorrhage is detected. Keep shock blocks near the foot end of the bed ready incase of necessity. When the patient is received in bed, cover with cover sheet except at the site where it must be folded back. Place a bed cradle over the stump to relieve the pressure of the top clothes. Use hot water bottles or radiant heat (heat cradle) to supply warmth to the limb.

Cardiac Bed

- Prepare the bed as open bed.
- Place back rest at the patient' s back making it comfortable with pillows and adjust according to the need of the patient
- Keep air cushion under the buttocks, a pillow under the knees and support the feet with foot rest board.
- Place the cardiac table in front of the patient with a pillow on it so that he or she can lean forward to rest his or her head and arms on it when gets tired in upright position. N.B: In acute heart disease, the patient is best nursed in flat position and in a chronic heart disease if there is difficulty in breathing the patient must be nursed in an upright position.

Blanket Bed

- Prepare the bottom of bed as open bed.
- Place long protective sheet and bed sheet over the bottom sheet and then arrange a small protective sheet and draw sheet in the usual manner.
- Arrange the electric blanket as per direction on the product, allow it to warm. If electric blanket is not available, arrange two or more ordinary woolen blankets on bed sheet and then arrange the top clothes.
- Arrange pillows or sand bags covered with

drawsheet after receiving the patient in bed (dressed in woolen clothes) to support the limbs steadily in case of arthritis for providing a comfortable position.

- Place bed cradle to take the weight of the top clothes off the painful joints.
- Provides extra warmth by using hot water bottles or radiant heat (heat cradle) to warm the patient, if necessary.

Burn Bed

- Repeat the steps as mentioned above in the preparation of open bed. Cover the mattress completely with long protective sheet. If mattress is without protective cover and then place sterile bottom sheet.
- Place three sterile draw sheets (top, middle and bottom) over the sterile bottom sheet and nicely tuck them under the mattress. These are helpful to permit changing by the nurse with minimal discomfort to the patient.

  In well established institutions microdon (3 M.co.) sheeting is used over the sterile bottom sheet. This prevents the patient from sticking to the sheet as a result of the exudate' s oozing from the burn area.
- Place the bed cradle over the burn area after receiving the patient in bed. Place a sterile sheet on the top and then cover with top clothes as in plaster bed. This prevents the patient from sticking to the sheets and helps to take the weight of top clothes off the burn area.

- Discard dirty and soiled linen in the dirty linen receptacle.
- Replace the locker. Dust the chair and stool and replace them also. Wash the duster, dry and replace it.
- Wash your hands.

CARE OF THE SKIN

The skin is an active organ with the functions of protection, secretion, excretion, temperature regulation and sensation. The skin has three primary layers; epidermis, dermis and subcutaneous. Bacteria commonly reside on the skin' s outer surface.

Normal skin Characteristics

- Skin is smooth and dry.
- Skin is intact and has no abrasion.
- Skin feels warm when palpated.
- The skin is soft and flexible.
- The skin is generally smooth and soft with good turgor (Elastic and Firm).
- Skin colour varies from deep brown to light pink

The Purposes of Bathing

- To keep the patient clean and comfortable and refreshed.
- To give a sense of well-being.
- To promote rest and sleep
- To keep the skin dry, active and healthy

Risk Factors for Skin Impairment

- Reduced sensation
- Poor nutrition
- Dehydration or oedema
- Excessive secretions and excretions on the skin.
- Vascular insufficiency.
- Use of external devices eg. cast, bandage or orthopedic devices.

Common Skin Problems

- Dry skin (flaky, rough, texture on exposed areas such as hands, arms, legs or face)
- Skin rashes results from overexposure to sunlight or moisture or from allergic reaction.
- Contact dermatitis: inflammation of the skin with scaly oozing lesions.

- Abrasion scrapping away of epidermis results in localized bleeding.
- Bacterial breakdown of sebum appears on face, neck, shoulders and back.

BED BATH

Definition Bathing the patient while he is in bed.
Purpose

- To cleanse the skin and thus increase elimination through it.
- To stimulate circulation through slightly active or entirely passive exercise
- To refresh the patient by relieving fatigue and discomfort.

General Instructions

- The temperature of the water should be 105o - 110oF (40o - 44°C)
- The water should be changed when it is cool or soapy.
- Be sure to remove all the soap as it is irritating to the skin
- Do not expose the patient unnecessarily
- Observe the patient's skin while bathing. Particularly if it is the first bath after admission. It offers an opportunity for the nurse to observe any rashes or pressure sores.

Equipment

- Mackintosh (long) and two bed sheets
- Soap in a soap tray
- Two sponging pads
- Towel - one
- Linen to change (Gown)
- Two jugs containing hot and cold water
- Basin
- Bucket
- Screen

- Urinal and bed pan

Procedure:

- Close the window or door and screen the bed to prevent draught and to avoid exposure.
- To collect the equipment next to the patients bed.
- And arrange the items conveniently at the bedside.
- Explain the procedure to the patient and get his cooperation
- Protect the bed with mackintosh and sheet
- Remove the patients linen and cover the patient
- Take water in the basin and feel with the back of your hand. The temperature should be comfortably hot.
- With wet sponge pad, moisten the patient' s face first.
- Apply soap. Carefully wash patient' s face, ears, and front of the neck. Dry with the towel. 10) Wash the left hand first and the right hand. Support patient' s arm by holding the wrist. Wash well between fingers if desired. The patient may place hands in basin.
- Remove the sheet up to the waist, ask the patients to keep the arms above his head. It will be easy to clean the axillae in this position. Clean chest and abdomen.
- Change water and turn the patient to the side and sponge his back. Give long firm strokes from back of neck to the buttocks. Watch for any redness over the pressure areas.
- Do the left leg first and then the right. Have the patient' s knee flexed so to facilitate washing. Give the bedpan and ask the patient to clean the genitals. If the patient is unable to do help to do it for him. Patient should be given privacy during this.
- The back care is done by applying alcohol, massage back, use long firm strokes starting form back of the neck out over the shoulders and down to the buttocks.

  Use also rotatory motion to increase the blood circulation. Extra attention to be given to the pressure areas

- Apply powder if indicated. This depends upon the condition of the skin. If the skin is wrinkled the application of powder is not advisable.
- If the patient is having dribbling of urine, zinc cream is applied.
- Role up the mackintosh and sheet when the patient is on the side. Then remove it from the other side. Put the soiled linen in the receptacle.
- Dress up the patient and remove the top sheet.
- The bed is tidied.
- The patient is given a warm drink
- Remove the articles from the bedside.
- Clean and replace in respective places.
- Send soiled linen for wash

Types of Therapeutic Baths

- Hot water tub bath: Immersion in hot water helps relieve muscle soreness and spasm. Water temperature should be 45° to 46°C.
- *Warm water tub bath*: Bathing in warm water relieves muscle tension. Water temperature should be 43°C.
- Cool water bath: Bathing in tipid water helps to lower body temperature when the body temperature is over 40°C (104°F). Water temperature should be 37°C.
- Sitz Bath:

Sitz Bath

Cleanses and reduces inflammation of the perineal and anal areas of a patient who has undergone rectal or perineal surgery or in hemorrhoids or fissures. Water temperature should be 43°C to 45°C.

Cold Sitz Bath

Cold sitz bath is more effective in relieving pain in the postoperative period.

- Back rub or back massage promotes relaxation, relieves, muscular tension and stimulates skin circulation. An effective back rub takes 3-5 minutes.

Care of Pressure Points and Prevention of Decubitus Ulcer

Prevention of decubitus ulcer in their patients who are bedridden is a major responsibility of nurses working in a hospital.

When we walk or stand on our two feet, the weight of our body is borne by our feet. But when an individual is confined to bed, the weight of his body has to be borne by his back or sides.

The skin of the soles of our feet is very tough and thick and it does not break easily in spite of the entire weight of the body being supported by it. The nature has designed the sole of the skin for weight bearing whereas the skin over the back of the body is not. When there is pressure on the skin of the back because of the weight of the body, the skin breaks and an ulcer develops.

Definition of Decubitus Ulcer

A decubitus ulcer is a pressure sore resulting from prolonged confinement in bed. Areas which are likely to be affected. When a patient lies in supine position, the following areas are vulnerable to pressure sores. Back of head Shoulder blades Elbows Base of the spine Buttocks Heels When a patient is in lateral position the following areas will be affected. Edge of ear Shoulders Knees Ankles All or any of the protuberant parts of a bedridden patient may become liable to pressure sores.

Causes of Decubitus Ulcer

Local or external causes 263 (a) Pressure: When any body prominence presses upon the bed, the tissues lying between them, get reduced blood supply - If this condition prolongs, the superficial tissues necrosed, skin breaks down and formation of an ulcer takes place.

The Following Conditions Cause Prolonged Pressure

- Leaving a patient in one position for a long time.
- Leaving a patient on a bedpan for a long while.

- Hard and lumpy mattress
- Pressure exerted by splints and plaster casts.
  - Friction:
- Friction from bedclothes or any other cause irritates the skin leading to inflammation.
- If you lie on a bed sheet, which has a rough seam in the middle of it, for a while, you will notice the impression of the seam on your back.
- You will also experience burning sensation and the part will be red in colour.

The Following Factors cause Friction in a Patient

- Careless pulling of patient and his linen
- Giving and removing bed pan carelessly
- Leaving broad crumbs, orange seeds and food particles on the bed
- Creases in the bottom sheet
- General restlessness of patient
- Rubbing two skin surfaces together
  - *Moisture:* Moisture makes the skin swollen, unhealthy and easily breakable.

The Following Reasons Eesult in Moisture over the Pressure Areas

Incontinence of faces and urine Severe perspiration Leaving a patient in wet linen

- *Heat:* Leaving a patient in one position for a long time, the part gets heated.
- Lack of cleanliness and irritating substances on the skin. e.g. perspiration, faeces, urine and vaginal discharge.

Predisposing Factor for Decupitus Ulcer

- Unconscious, helpless or acutely ill patients These patients are unable to appreciate the weight of pressure and change their positions
- Paralysed patients (Paraplegic and quadriplegic patients). They have lost motor and sensory functions.

- Patients with incontinence (spinal injuries)
- Old people
- Very emaciated and malnourished people
- Patients with dehydration or oedema
- Very fat people
- Patients with disease affecting circulation e.g. heart diseases and anemia
- Patients with debilitating diseases such as cancer and tuberculosis j. Patients with metabolic disorders. eg.

Diabetes Prevention of Decubitus Ulcers

Prevent Pressure

- Establish a turning schedule for bedridden patients; turn hourly.
- Have a firm cot and foam mattress for bed-ridden patients - use extra pillows, pads and air rings to reduce pressure.

Prevent Friction

- When changing position of your patient lift him and do not drag him on to bed. 265
- Keep sheets without wrinkles and seams.
- Keep bed clean and free from crumbs.
- If patient is restless, protect pressure points with soft pads.

Prevent Moisture

- Keep dressings and bed dry and clean.
- Clean and dry the incontinent patients promptly.
- Prevent predisposing causes:
  - Improve patient's health by means of good food, ventilation, sunlight and exercises.
  - Encourage circulation through massage.
  - Have patient to ambulate early.
- Observe early signs and symptoms of decubitus ulcers:
  - Redness

- Dark discoloration.
- Bruising,
- Tenderness of the area.
- Burning sensation.

- Give good care to pressure points: Careful cleaning and massage should be carried out 3 or 4 times a day for all bedridden patients. For some patients, it is necessary to give care as often as every two hours.
  - Equipment A bowl of warm water Sponge cloth Soap Towel Dusting powder Spirit
  - Procedure Explain procedure to patient - Arrange articles at the bedside. Screen the bed Wet the part with soapy hand massage the area in circular movements, so that the tissues under the skin gets increased circulation Remove soap by washing Dry the areas Apply spirit over the area and massage well. Spirit helps to harden the skin. Apply lightly dusting powder to keep the part thoroughly dry. Do this treatment to all pressure points. If patient is incontinent, apply zinc cream instead of spirit and powder. This protects the skin from moisture. Leave patient comfortable after the procedure.

Treatment of Decubitus Ulcer

- Clean ulcers with aseptic precautions - Use antiseptics such as eusole or hydrogen peroxide.
- Apply medication ordered by the doctor. eg. Antibiotic ointment, shark liver oil, zinc oxide, or any other topical applications.
- Cover with sterile dressings and bandage
- Surgical fermentation, ultraviolet rays or heat lamp are helpful in healing
- Provide good nutrition
- Prevent secondary infections.

CARE OF THE FEET AND NAILS

The feet and nails require special attention to prevent

infection, odors, and an injury to tissue. People are unaware of foot or nail problems until pain or discomfort occurs. Problems may result from poor care of the feet and nails such as biting nails or trimming them improperly, exposure to chemicals and wearing poorly fitted shoes.

Purposes of care of the nails

- To keep nails harmless
- To prevent accumulation of dirt under the nails and reduce occurrence of infection

Characteristics of a healthy nail

A normal healthy nail is transparent, smooth and convex with pink nail beds and translucent white tips.

Care of nail and foot

- Inspect the feet daily including the tops and soles of the feet and the area between the toes.
- Wash and soak the feet daily using luke warm water (37°C).
- F the feet perspire, apply a bland foot powder.
- If dryness is noted along the feet, apply soft oil and rub gently into the skin.
- File the toe nails straight across and square.
- Avoid wearing elastic stockings.
- Wear clean socks daily.
- Do not walk barefoot.
- Wear properly fitted shoes.
- Exercise regularly to improve circulation to the lower extremities. 1
- Immediately wash minor cuts and dry them thor oughly. Mild anticeptics may be applied to the skin,

Risk Factors for foot and nail Ailments

- Patients with peripheral vascular disease eg. Diabetes mellitus.
- Patients with neuropathy (degeneration of peripheral nerves characterized by loss of sensation)

- Poor ill fitting foot wear
- Poor knowledge of foot and nail care

Common foot and Nail Problems

- *Callus:* Is a thickened portion of epidermis caused by local friction or pressure.
- *Corns:* Is caused by friction and pressure from shoes. It is seem mainly on toes, over bony prominence.
- Plantar warts are fungating lesions, appearing on sole of foot and is caused by Papilloma virus.
- Athlete' s foot (Tinea pedis) is the fungal infection of foot mainly induced by wearing of constricting footwear.
- *Ingrown nails:* Toenails or finger nails grow inward into soft tissue around nail resulting from improper nail trimming.
- Paronychia is the inflammation of tissue surrounding nails following an injury. It is common among diabetic patients.
- Foot odor or result of excessive perspiration promoting micro organism growth.

Equipment

A tray containing

- A pair of scissors or a nail clipper
- Wet swabs in a small bowl
- A jug with water for washing hands
- A kidney tray with dettol 1 in 40 solution
- Soft nail brush
- A paper bag
- A towel.

Procedure

- Assemble articles at the bed side of the patient.
- Explain the procedure to the patient and get his cooperation.
- Place towel under the hands.
- Wash hands of patient with soap and water. Use

brush if the nails are very dirty. Soak nails in water to cut them easily.

- Cut finger nails to the shape of the nails. Cut toe nails straight across to prevent in- growing toe nails. Take care not to injure the flesh.
- Receive soiled wipers in the paper bag.
- Wash hands and dry.
- Clean and sterilize nail clipper/scissors and replace in their proper place.
- Dispose off soiled wipers with the paper bag.

ORAL HYGIENE

The Oral cavity is lined with mucous membrane continuous with the skin. The mucuous membrane is an epithelial tissue that lines and protects organs, secretes mucous to keep passageways of digestive system moist and lubricated, and absorbs nutrition.

Purposes of Oral Hygiene

- Oral improve taste

Proper Oral Hygiene

- Good oral hygiene involves cleanliness, comfort and the moisturizing the mouth structures. Proper care prevents oral disease and tooth destruction.
- Brushing, flossing and irrigation are necessary for proprer cleansing.
- To prevent tooth decay, reduces the intake of carbohydrates, especially sweet snacks between meals.
- Brushing of the teeth atleast four times a day is a basic to an effective oral hygiene(after meals and at bed time)
- Tooth brushes should be replaced every three months
- After brushing,thorough rinsing is important to remove dislodged food particles

Risk Factors for Oral Problems

- Patients who are paralyzed or seriously ill.

- Unconscious patients
- Diabetic patients
- Patients undergoing radiation theraphy
- Patients receiving chemotheraphy
- Patients having oral surgery, trauma
- Patients with immunosuppression drug eg HIV patients

Common Oral Problems

The two major types of oral problems are dental caries (cavities) and periodontal disease (Pyorrhea)

- Dental caries is the most common oral problem of younger people. The development of the cavities involve the destruction of tooth enamel through decalcification. Decalcification is a result of an accumulation of mucin, carbohydrates and lactic acid bacilli in the saliva normally found in the mouth, which forms a coating on the teeth called plaque. Plaque is transparent and adheres to the teeth near the base of the crown at the gum margins. The plaque prevents normal acid dilution and neutralization, preventing the dissolution of bacteria in the oral cavity. The acid eventually destroys the tooth enamel and in severe cases, the pulp, or inner sponge tissue of the teeth.
- Periodontal disease is the disease of the tissue around the tooth. It is an inflammation of the periodontal membrane. It is the most common problem of people over 35 years of age. The calculus deposit on teeth at the gum line. The gingivae become swollen and tender. Then the inflammation spreads, pockets develop between gums and gingivae. The alveolar bone is destroyed and the teeth loosen.
- Halitosis (Bad breath) is a common problem of the oral cavity. Causes:
  - Poor oral hygiene
  - Inspection of the oral cavity
  - Liver disease–Diabetes

- Cheilosis is the disorder involves cracking of the lips especially at the ankle of the mouth. Causes:
  - Riboflavin deficiency
  - Mouth breathing
  - Excess salivation
- Stomatitis is an inflammative condition of the mouth. Causes:
  - Contact with irritants such as tobacco
  - Vitamin deficiency
  - Infection by bacteria, viruses or fungi
  - Use of Chemotherapeutic drugs
- Glossitis is an inflammation of the tongue resulting from an infectious disease or injury such as burn or bite.
- Gingivitis is a inflammation of the gums usually resulting from poor oral hygiene.
- Oral malignancies: lumps are ulcer appears in or around the mouth. The most common site is at the base of the tongue. Causes:
  - Pipe smoking
  - Tobacco chewing

Equipments: A tray Containing

- Cotton swab or clean linen pieces in a bowl
- Forceps (artery and dissecting forceps)
- Gallicups 2 nos. (one for Glycering borax another for salt solution)
- Feeding cup with salt solution
- Kidney trays 2
- Swabs sticks
- Rubber sheet
- Towel
- Wash towel

Procedure

- Place all the articles at conveniently on the bedside table.
- Explain the procedure to the patient
- Put the rubber sheet (mackintosh) with towel and kidney tray under the chin

- Have the patient rinsed his mouth with salt solution form the feeding cup
- Turn the patient' s head to one side
- Take the artery forceps, wrap a piece of linen around the tip of the forceps
- Dip it inside the saline water and clean the teeth with up and down movements.
- Pay special attention to inside the mouth, gums, inside the cheeks, tongue and the roof of the mouth
- Change linen pieces as often as necessary.
- Discard used cotton in the other kidney tray
- Allow the patient to gargle as much as necessary
- Dip the swap stick in glycerin borax, swab gums, root and sides of the mouth.

After Care of Equipments

- Clean kidney trays and feeding cups with soap and water.
- Boil forceps, and gallicups after cleaning
- Place all articles in their places after cleaning and boiling.

Care of Dentures

If the patient has dentures, care should taken to keep the dentures clean. If the patient is unable to do so, the nurse has to remove the dentures by grasping it with gauze pieces, place them in a tumbler or cup containing water. Dentures are washed carefully busing brush, toothpaste and cool water. Water, which is too hot, may injure the composition of dentures. If the patient is to do by himself, he may be assisted. Remove dentures of patients who are unconscious, mentally ill and who have vomiting or cough spasm

CARE OF THE HAIR

Care of the hair is a part of daily hygiene. A person's appearance and a feeling of well-being depend on the way the hair looks and feels, hair growth, distribution and pattern can be indicators of general health status.

Proper Hair Care

- Frequent brushing helps keep hair clean and distributes oil evenly along hair shafts
- Short-tooth combs are adequate for short hairs
- Large-tooth combs are preferable for curly hair
- Avoid using combs with sharp and irregular teeth

Factors that Affect the Character of Hair

- Hormonal changes
- Emotional and physical stress
- Ageing
- Infection 274
- Certain diseases like cancer
- Certain drugs like chemotherapy.

Common Hair and Scalp Problems:

- *Dandruff*: dandruff is the scaling of scalp accompanied by itching. In severe cases, dandruff is found on eyebrows
- *Pediculosis* (*lice*): tiny grayish-white parasite insects infest human beings
- *Pediculosis capitis* (*head lice*): parasite is found on scalp attached to hair strands
- *Pediculosis corporis* (*body lice*): parasites cling to clothing and sucks blood
- *Pediculosis pubis* (*crab lice*): parasites are found in pubic hair
  - Hair loss (alopecia)

Purposes:

- To maintain cleanliness
- To prevent matting
- To promote comfort
- To remove dirt and dandruff by combing and brushing
- To give exercise to scalp
- To get an opportunity to examine the scalp and the hair of patients who are acutely ill
- To soothen the patient and to help induce sleep.

Equipment A tray containing the following articles to be taken to the bedside.

- Brush and comb
- A little oil in a small bottle
- Kidney tray with 1 in 40 dettol solution
- Cotton swabs (wet)
- Ribbon
- Towel

Procedure

- Arrange articles at the right side of the patient
- Explain the procedure to the patient and get her cooperation
- Get the patient to sit up if her condition permits
- Place a towel around the shoulders to prevent soiling her bed clothes
- Smear your finger with oil and apply on the scalp and hair
- Massage scalp in a circular movement to promote good circulation
- Brush and comb hair free from tangles. Take a few strands of hair at a time.
  Hold it with your left hand tightly at the root of the hair to prevent pulling of hair and comb it from top to downwards. Wipe the comb with a wet swab and examine for pediculi. Dispose of soiled swabs in a paper bag.
- Braid the hair and tie with ribbon.
- Keep patient comfortable and clean and put away the equipment.

ATTENDING HAIR CARE WASHING PURPOSE

- To keep the hair clean and healthy.
- To prevent itching, infection infestation.
- To provide a sense of well being.
- To destroy pediculi.

SUPPLIES

- Combing - hair oil, comb and paper bag.

- Washing
  - A tray containing
- Hot and cold water in jugs.
- ·A basin and a mug.
- Protective sheets- two, one large and one small.
- A piece of bandage.
- Soap/shampoo.
- Little cotton in bowl.
- Wash cloth.
- Bath towel.
- Hot water bottle with cover.
  - Bucket - one N.B. Make a trough of large protective sheet with a piece of bandage rolled in it.
- Treating pediculosis
  - Pediculosis capits (Head louse)
- A gown for the nurse.
- A tray containing
  - Fine tooth comb
  - Parasiticide
  - Antiseptic lotion in a kidney tray and paper bag.
  - Supplies for washing hair in bed (as above) incase patient is bedridden.
  - Pediculosis corporis or vestimenti(Body louse) - Refer Antiseptic Bath in procedure "Appling Hot Applications".
  - Pediculosis pubis (Crab louse)
- A tray containing
  - Protective sheet and towel.
  - Bowl of warm water.
  - Razor and blade.
  - Soap and brush.
  - Antiseptic lotion in a kidney tray and paper bag.
- Forceps to pick up lice from eye brows and eyelashes.

Guidelines

- Combing Hair are combed and arranged in the style the patient prefers at least twice a day.
- When washing the hair, follow as under

- The patients are given hair wash at least once a week and bedridden patients are given hair wash in bed.
- Avoid hair wash for the patient who has just taken meals atleast for an hour.
- Avoid exposure and chilling by

- Keeping the patient covered with top clothes.
- Closing the windows and doors of the room.
- Keeping the room warm.
- Finishing the hair wash quickly.
  - If the patient is very sick, note pulse before and after the hair wash.
  - Do not let the patient exert. Try to avoid exertion to the patient as far as possible.
- When treating pediculosis, nurse must have following information.
  - The pediculi are small, grey coloured, blood sucking parasites which live for several days in the hair. The female lays about 50 eggs/nits which are grey or white in colour, cling to hair and hatch in about one week.
  - The symptoms of pediculi are
- Itching
- Scalp, neck and behind ears in head louse.
- All over the body in body louse.
- On and around the part affected in crab louse.
- Rash
- Neck and behind ears in head louse
- All over the body in body louse.
- On and around the part affected in crab louse.
- Sores
- Scalp in head louse.
- Body in body louse.
- On the part affected in crab louse.
- Restlessness and irritability
  - The common parasiticides used are
- Mediker
- Cyban

Nursing Activity

- Wash your hands and put on gown.
- Take supplies to the bedside.
- Maintain privacy by using screen.
- Explain the procedure to the patient.
- Give hair care.
  - Combing
- Loosen the hair.
- Apply oil to hair if necessary.
- Comb and arrange the hair in the style the patient prefers.
- If hair are braided, secure the end of braid.
- Replace the supplies.
  - Washing
- Position the patient bringing head on the edge of bed and shoulders raised on a pillow so that head is slightly down. " Place the protective sheet and bath towel under the head.
- Place the trough in the patient' s neck and direct it into the bucket.
- Place cotton in patient' s ears and wash cloth over eyes.
- Loosen the hair and remove hair pins
- Mix hot and cold water and check the temperature of water at the back of hand.
- Wet the hair, apply soap and shampoo and work up the lather.
- Start cleaning at the hairline and work towards the back of the head and then to the front of head symmetrically. Message the scalp first and then the hair with the finger tips. Add water as necessary to work up the lather.
- Rinse thoroughly. Squeeze off water from the hair.
- Wrap bath towel around the hair.
- Remove the trough and slip the pillow under the head by raising head and shoulder. Place patients head on protective sheet over the pillow and rub the head gently with towel. Spread the hair out on bath

towel with hot water bottle underneath to dry in winter.

- When it is dry, apply oil, comb it arrange in the style the patient prefers.
- Remove, clean,dry, and replace the supplies.
  - Treating pediculosiss
- Prediculsis capits (head louse)
  - Put on gown and follow first five steps a of washing.
  - Wet the hair, pour mediker on hair, massage the scalp first and then the hair with finger tips working from the hairline towards the back and then the front of the head symmetrically. Add water as necessary to work up the lather. Leave the hair in lather for five minutes and rinse.
  - Follow the procedure mentioned above.
  - Repeat the treatment within few days.
  - Remove the supplies, wash and boil the supplies soak gown, clothes and linen in carbolic solution 1:20 for four hours before sending to laundary.
  - Soak comb and protective sheet in above solution for hours, then wash and dry.
- Pediculosis corporis/ vestimenti (Body louse)
- Five a disinfectant bath.
- Apply antiseptic ointment to heal any injuries produced by scatching.
- Ffollow steps iv and v as above.
- Pediculosis pubes (crab louse)
- The hair of affected areas (pubes or axilllae) shaved and burnt.
- Apply disinfectant into the areas and after some hours patient given bath.
- In case eyebrows and eyelashes are affected, pick up lice with forceps and apply two per cent of yellow oxide of mercury.
- Follow step iii as above.
- Wash your hands thoroughly.

Recording Record in the nurse' s notes as under.

- Combing any dandruff, pediculosis or anyother abnormal condition regarding hair or scalp.
- Washing time of giving hair wash, soap, shampoo used, patients reaction.
- Treating pediculosis The time, parasisticide used and the effect of treatment.

CARE OF EYES,EARS AND NOSE: EYES

Normally no special care is required for the eyes because they are continually cleansed by tears, and the eyelids and the lashes prevent the entrance of foreign particles. a person needs only to remove any dried secretions that have collected on the inner canthus or the eyelashes.

Unconscious clients are at risk for eye injury because the blink reflex may be absent. In these clients, excessive drainage frequently collects along eyelid margins. Special attentions are also needed for clients who have had eye surgery or an eye infection.

That can result in increased discharge or drainage. The nurse often assists clients in the care of eyeglasses, contact lenses, or artificial eyes.

EARS

Hygiene of the ears has implications for hearing acuity when wax or foreign substances collect in the external ear canal, and they interfere with sound conduction. Older adults are particularly susceptible to this problem.

The nurse should be sensitive to any behavioral cues that might indicate a hearing impairment. When caring for a client with the hearing aid the nurse instructs the client on proper cleansing and maintenance as well as communication techniques, that promote hearing the spoken words.

NOSE

- The nose provides for the sense. It also controls the temperature and humidity of inhaled air. It also prevents entrance of foreign particles into the respiratory system.

- The accumulation of encrusted secretions within the nose can impair olfactory sensation and breathing. Irritation of nasal mucosa can cause swelling leading to obstruction. Hygiene care of the nose is simple.

Clients who need special care

- Pateints with naso gastric tube feeding
- Patients with the endotracheal tubes

Chapter 7

Health Assessments

Health assessment is an important component in health care for proper diagnosis and effective treatment. Health assessment includes the following:

- Physical assessment
- Head to foot examination
- Systemwise examination
- Recording height and weight,
- Mental status examination
- Laboratory investigation
- Special investigation

TECHNIQUES IN PHYSICAL ASSESSMENT

Techniques in physical assessment are

- *Inspection:* It means looking with eyes. It reveals any rash scar, colour, size shape, contour and symmetry of the body parts
- *Palpation:* It means feeling using sense of touch. It reveals any swelling, coldness, hotness, stiffness, hardness, smoothness, roughness, pain, vibration, firmness and flaccidity
- *Percussion:* It means striking or tapping with fingers. It elicits sounds which indicate whether the underlined tissues are solid or filled with fluid.

The Sounds May Vary

- *Resonant:* A loud sound over the normal lung tissue
- *Tympanic:* A drum like sound over the air filled tissues such as gastric air bubble.
- *Dull:* A medium pitched sound with medium

duration without resonance, heard over the solid tissues, such as heart, liver.

- *Flat:* A pitched sound with short duration without resonance, heard over the complete solid tissues, such as bones.

- *Auscultation:* It means listen with stethoscope or placing the ear against the body. It reveals sounds produced within the body and the blood vessels such as heart beat, bowel sounds.
- *Manipulation:* It means moving with the body parts. It reveals rigidity, difficulty or discomfort in moving the body parts.
- *Reflex testing:* Means automatic response to a given stimulus. It reveals reflex is present, or not present, strength and movements of hands and legs.
- Olfaction: It means sense of smell (odour). It reveals the nature of disease condition of the patient.

TAKING HEIGHT AND WEIGHT

It is a measurement from head to toe that indicates the state of growth and health. It is measured in feet, inches or centimeters.

Purpose

- To measure accurate height of the patients

Equipments

- Measuring scale attached to the wall
- A straight object
- Paper and pencil
- Newspaper

Guidelines

- Have the patient' s shoes/ slippers removed while taking height to avoid any variations in the reading
- If thick object is placed on the top of the head, at right angle to the scale indicating the reading, note the bottom reading of the object.

Procedure

- Gather the equipments
- Explain the purpose and the procedure to the patient

- Wash your hands
- Tell the patient to remove the slippers or shoes
- Assist the patient to stand on a lean newspaper kept on the floor.
- Tell the patient to stand with the buttocks and the back of head against the scale on wall, feet flat, heals together and eyes looking straight ahead.
- Place the straight object on the top of the head at right angles to the scale on wall, touching the scale calibration. Note the reading where the said object touches the scale
- Tell the patient to put on slippers.
- Place the patient in a comfortable position.
- Replace the equipments.
- Wash your hands.
- Record the date and time of the procedure and the height in the nurse' s notes or graphic sheet Taking weight It is the quantitative expression of a body that indicate the state of growth and health It is measured in kilograms, pounds or grams

Purposes

- To obtain accurate weight of the patient
- To aid in accurate diagnosis of the patient
- To evaluate patient' s response to treatment

Equipments

- Weighing scale
- Newspaper

Guidelines

- Weigh on weighing scale when the patient is ambulatory
- Sdaily weigh the patient at the same time with the same scale and with same clothing
- Weigh before meals and after voiding
- Weigh on admission to provide a base line information to subsequent daily weight recording and assess any significant increase or decrease in the patient' s weight.
- The weighing scale must be accurate, hence the

balance scale, be prepared before weighing the patient

Procedure

- Gather the equipments
- Explain the purpose and procedure to the patient
- Wash your hands
- Assist the patient to void or empty the bladder.
- Check the commonly used flat weighing machine' s reading is set at zero level.
- Tell the patient to remove the slippers or shoes and extra clothes.
- Assist the patient to step on the centre of the scale platform.
- Assist the patient to step off the scale platform.
- Assist the patient to return to the bed
- Wash your hands
- Record the weight in the graphic sheet or nurse' s notes.

VITAL SIGNS

The importance of vital sign in health sciences Vital signs include the physiological measurements of temperature, Pulse, BP and respirations. Vital signs are a quick and efficient way of monitoring a patient' s condition or identifying problems and evaluating the patient' s response to intervening changes. One vital sign can influence characteristics of other vital signs. The basic techniques of inspection, palpation and auscultation are used to determine vital signs.

Assessment of vital signs allows the nurse to identify nursing diagnoses, to implement planned intervention and to evaluate success. When the nurse learns the physiological variables influencing vital signs and recognizes the relationship of vital sign changes to other physiological assessment findings, precise determination of the client' s health problems can be made.

Vital signs and normal ranges for adults

- Temperature 36° to 38°C (96.4 to 98.6 F)
- Pulse 60 – 100 beats/mt

- Respiration 12–20 breaths/mt
- Blood pressure Average 120/80 mmHg

Guidelines for Assessing Vital Signs

- The nurse caring for the patient is responsible for assessing vital signs. The nurse should obtain the vital signs, interpret their significance and make decisions about interventions.
- Equipment used to measure vital signs must work properly to ensure accurate findings.
- Equipment should be selected based on the client's condition and characteristics.
- The nurse controls or minimizes environmental factors that may affect vital signs.
- The nurse uses an organized, systematic approach when taking vital signs. Each procedure requires a step-by-step approach to ensure accuracy.
- The manner of approach to the patient can alter the vital signs. The nurse should approach the patient in a calm caring manner while taking vital signs.
- Based on patient' s condition, the nurse collaborates with the physician to decide the frequency of vital signs assessment.
- The nurse analyzes the results of vital signs measurement. The nurse is often in the best position to assess all clinical finding about a patient.
- The nurse verifies and communicates significant changes in vital signs. The nurse informs the physician of abnormal vital signs.
- Vital signs are documented and communicated to the nurse assuming care of the patient and well of patient.

Body Temperature

- Temperature is the "hotness" or "coldness" of a substance.
- Body temperature is the difference between the amount of heat produced by body processes and the

amount of heat lost to the external environment. Heat produced - Heat lost = Body temperature.

- Normal body temperature: For healthy young adults the average body temperature is 37°C (98.6°F). The body tissues and cells function best in the normal body temperature.
- Core temperature is temperature of deep tissues. Despite extreme in environmental condition and physical activity, the temperature - control mechanisms of the human beings maintains the body' s core temperature constant. Surface temperature fluctuates depending on blood flow to the skin and the amount of heat lost to the external environment.

Temperature: control mechanism of human beings The body temperature is precisely regulated by physiological and behavioral mechanisms.

For body temperature to stay constant and with normal range, the relationship between heat production and heat loss must be maintained. The relationship is regulated by neurological and cardiovascular mechanisms. The nurse applies knowledge of temperature control mechanisms to promote temperature regulation.

Neural and Vascular Control

- The hypothalamus located between the cerebral hemispheres, controls the body temperature.
- The hypothalamus senses main changes in body temperature.
- The anterior hypothalamus controls the heat production.
- A comfortable temperature is the "set point" at which a heating system operates.
- When the nerve cells in the anterior hypothalamus became heated beyond the set point, impulses are sent out to reduce body temperature.
- Mechanisms of heat loss include sweating, vasodilatation (widing) of blood vessels and inhibition of heat production.

- If the posterior hypothalamus senses the body temperature is lower than the set point, heat conservation mechanisms are instituted.
- Vasoconstrction (narrowing of blood vessels) reduces blood flow to the skin and extremities.
- Heat production is stimulated through voluntary muscle contraction and muscle shivering.
- Trauma to the hypothalamus or to the spinal cord (which carries hypothalamic tract) can cause serious alternations in temperature control.

Heat production

Thermoregulation requires the normal function of heat - production processes. Heat is produced in the body by metabolism which is the chemical reaction in all body cells. Activities requiring additional chemical reactions increase the metabolic rate.

As metabolism increases additional heat is produced. When metabolism decreases, less heat is produced. Heat production occurs during rest, voluntary movements and involuntary shivering.

(shivering is an involuntary body response to temperature differences in the body). Shivering can increase heat production 4 to 5 times greater than normal. Heat is produced to equalize body temperature. Heat loss Heat production and heat loss occur simultaneously. The skin' s structure and exposure to the environment result in constant, normal heat loss through reduction, conduction, convection and evaporation.

- Radiation is the transfer of heat from the surface of another without actual contact between the two. Peripheral vasodilatation increases blood flow to the skin to increase heat loss. Peripheral vasoconstriction minimizes blood flow to the skin and inhibits heat loss.
- Conduction is the transfer of heat from one object to another with direct contact.
- Convection is the transfer of heat away by air movement. Heat is first conducted to air molecules

directly in contact with the skin. Air current carry away the warmed air.

- Evaporation is the transfer of heat energy when a liquid is changed to a gas. The body continuously losses heat by evaporation. About 600 - 900 ml of water evaporates from skin and lungs daily, resulting in water and heat loss.

  By regulating sweating, the body promotes additional evaporation and heat loss. When body temperature rises, the anterior hypothalamus signals the sweat glands to release sweat to evaporate from the skin surface, resulting in heat loss. Factors affecting body temperature.

  Many factors affect body temperature. The nurse must be aware of these factors when assessing temperature variables and evaluating deviation from normal.

- *Age:* For new born, the temperature - control mechanisms are immature. An infant' s temperature may respond drastically to changes in the environment.

  Temperature regulation is unstable until children reach puberty. Older adults are sensitive to temperature extremes because of deterioration in control mechanisms, reduced sweat gland activity, reduced amounts of subcutaneous fat and reduced metabolism.

- Exercise: Muscle activity causes increased metabolism by increasing carbohydrate and fat breakdown. Any form of exercise can increase heat production and thus body temperature.
- *Hormone level:* Women generally experience greater fluctuations in body temperature than men. Hormonal variations during menstrual cycle cause body temperature fluctuation. Temperature changes occur in women during menopause. (cessation of menstruation)
- *Circadian rhythm:* Body temperature normally changes

0.5° to 1°C during 24 hour period. The temperature is usually lowest between 1.00 AM and 4.00 AM.

- *Stress:* Physical and emotional stress increases body temperature through hormonal and neural stimulation.
  These physiological changes increase metabolism, which increases heat production.
- *Environment:* Environment influences body temperature in a very warm room, the body temperature will be elevated. In a cold weather, the body temperature may be low because of extensive radiant and conductive heat loss.
- *Temperature alterations*: Changes in body temperature can be related to excess heat production, excessive heat loss, minimal heat production, minimal heat loss or any combination of these.
- *Fever:* Hyperpyrexia or fever occurs because heat loss mechanisms are unable to keep pace with excess heat production, resulting in an abnormal rise in body temperature.
- *Hyperpyrexia:* An elevated body temperature related to the body' s inability to promote heat loss or reduce heat production is hyperthermia. Any disease or trauma to the hypothalamus can impair heat loss mechanisms.
- *Heat stroke:* Prolonged exposure to the sun or high environmental temperature can overwhelm the body' s heat loss mechanisms. Heat also depresses hypothalamic function.
  These conditions cause heat stroke, a dangerous emergency condition with a high mortality rate. Patients at risk for heat stroke are the very young, very old, cardio vascular condition, diabetes and alcoholics.
- Hypothermia: Heat loss during prolonged exposure to cold overwhelms the body ability to produce heat causing hypothermia. Hypothermia is classified as follows:

Classification of Hypothermia

	Centigrade	Farenheit
Mild	33 – 36°F	91.4°– 96.8°
Moderate	30 – 33°	86.0°– 91.4°
Severe	27 – 30°	80.6°– 86.0°
Profound	< 30°	< 80.6°

Frost bits occurs when the body is exposed to subnormal temperature. Ice crystals farming inside the cell result in permanent circulatory and tissue damage. Areas at risk for frost bite are the carlobes, tip of the nose and fingers and toes. The injured area is white, waxy and firm to touch.

Sites for Assessing Temperature

- Oral
- Rectal
- Axillary
- Tympanic route

Types of Thermometers

- Mercury - in - glass thermometers
- Electronic thermometer
- Disposable thermometer

Purpose of Taking Temperature

- To aid in diagnosis or the patient' s condition
- To find out the progress of the patient

Taking Temperature by Mouth General Instructions

- Oral temperature should not be taken immediately after the patient has had a hot or a cold drink or food.
- Oral temperature should not be taken for the following patients
- Children below the age of five years opatients receiving oxygen
- Patients with nasal obstruction, dyspnoea or sore mouth

- Patient who are delirious, unconscious and not cooperating, hysterical, restless or mentally ill
- Patients with oral surgeries

Procedure (Recording temperature - oral) Equipment

Tray Containing

- 3 or 4 test tubes or bottles with antiseptic lotions savlon 2per cent) and a little cotton underneath
- A glass tumbler with clean water and little cotton underneath
- A bowl containing a bit soapy white wipers
- A small piece of clean cloth
- A kidney tray
- A paper bag
- watch with second hand
- Red lead pen

Procedure

- Explain the procedure and take the patients cooperation
- Let the patient be sitting or lying down
- Remove thermometer from the lotion, wash with clean water and dry with clean piece of cloth from the bulb upwards to prevent bacteria from setting down on the lower part which goes into the mouth of the patient.
- Shake down the mercury by a quick sudden movement of the wrist and bring down the mercury level at 95°f. Place the bulb of the thermometer under the tongue and tell the patient not to bite the thermometer but to hold it with his lips.
- Leave the thermometer in the mouth for 2 minutes (during this time take his pulse and respiration).
- Remove the thermometer, note the temperature clean with the soapy wiper from above downwards towards the bulb (to prevent bacteria from spreading all over the thermometer.
- Collect the dirty soapy water in the kidney tray and place the dirty wiper in the paper bag

- Replace thermometer in the test tube or bottle with the lotion
- Record the temperature in the chart

After care of the Equipment

- Clean all the articles used.
- Wash the thermometer with soap and cold water
- Keep the thermometer in the antiseptic lotion for 2 to 5 minutes
- Reset the tray and keep it ready for the next use.

Nursing care of Individual with Altered body Temperature Hyperthermia

- Obtain all vital signs
- Observe skin colour
- Observe for shivering are diaphoresis

Non - pharmacological therapy

Non - pharmacological therapy are methods that increase heat loss by evaporation, convection conduction or reduction.

- Tepid sponge bathes
- Bathing with alcohol - water solution
- Cooling fans
- Allow rest period
- Limit physical activity
- Reduce external covering on patient' s body to promote heat
- Loss through reduction and conduction.
- Provide fluids (atleast 3 litres per day) to replace fluids loss.
- Encourage oral hygiene because oral mucous membranes dry easily from dehydration. 10) Provide measures to stimulate appetite and offer well balanced meals.
- Provide supplemental oxygen therapy as ordered to improve oxygen delivery to body cells.
- Control environmental temperature without inducing shivering. Eg. Cooling fans

Heat stroke

The best treatment for heat stroke is prevention. The nurse teaches the patient:

- To avoid strenuous work in hot weather.
- To drink fluids such as clear fruit juices before, during and after exercise.
- To wear loose cotton clothing.
- To avoid exercising in areas with poor ventilation.
- To wear protective hats over the head when going outdoors.

First aid for heat stroke

- Move the patient to cooler environment.
- Reduce clothing covering the body
- Place wet towel over the skin
- Use cooling fans to increase heat loss
- Summon emergency medical treatment (intravenous fluids)

Hypothermia

Prevention is the key for patient' s at risk for hypothermia and frostbite.

- Educate patient who are at risk for hypothermia (Eg. the very young, the very old, persons debilitated by trauma, stroke, diabetes, drug or alcohol intoxication, sepsis, mentally ill, alcohol intoxication, malnutrition). Treatment
- Prevent a further decrease in body temperature.
- Remove wet clothes, provide dry ones and wrap the client in blanket.
- If the patient is conscious offer warm liquids such as milk or soups
- Place the patient in a warm room
- When the patient reaches emergency treatment, patients are closely monitored for cardiac irregularities and electrolyte imbalances.

PULSE

The pulse is the palpable bounding of blood flow noted

at various points of body. pulse is an indicator of circulatory status. Circulation is the means by which cells receive nutrients and oxygen and remove waste products of metabolism. For cells to function normally, there must be a continuous blood flow and an appropriate volume and distribution of blood to cells that need nutrients. Blood flows through the body in a continuous circuit. Electrical impulses originating from the sinoatrial (SA) node travel through heart muscle to stimulate Cardiac contraction.

When, about 60 to 70 ml of blood enters aorta during each ventricular contraction the wall of aorta distends creating a pulse wave. This pulse wave travels rapidly toward the distal ends of arteries. When the pulse wave reaches a peripheral artery, it can be felt by palpating the artery lightly against underlying bone or muscle. The pulse is the palpable bounding of the blood flow in the peripheral artery. The pulse rate is the number of pulsing sensation occurring in one minute.

Assessment of pulse

Any artery can be assessed for pulse rate, but the radial and carotid arteries are easily palpated.

Peripheral pulse site

Character of the pulse

Assessment of radial pulse includes measurement of the rate, rhythm, strength and quality.

RATE Pulse rate is counted for minute when the patient is in a sitting, standing and lying position.

Normal heart rate

Age	*Heart rat*
Infant	120 – 160/min
Toddlers	90 – 140/ min
Pre Schooler	80 – 110/ min
School Going	75 – 100/ min
Adolescents	60 – 90/ min
Adult	60 – 100/ min

Factors influencing pulse rate

- *Exercise:* Short term exercise increases pulse rate. An athlete, who participates in long - term exercise will have lower pulse rate at rest.
- *Temperature:* Fever and heat increases pulse rate. Hypothermic decreases pulse rate.
- *Emotion:* Pain and anxiety increase pulse rate.
- *Drugs:* Epinephrine increases pulse rate.
- Digoxin decreases pulse rate.
- Hemorrhage: blood loss increases pulse rate
- *Postural changes:* In standing or sitting positions, pulse rate increases. In lying down position, the pulse rate decreases.
- *Pulmonary condition:* Causes poor oxygenation and decreased pulse rate.

Purposes of Monitoring Pulse

- To test the health and efficiency of heart
- To test the elasticity and the health of arteries.
- To get an approximately idea of how much blood is being pumped into the artery system.
- To estimate the change in the needs of the body circulation.
- To understand the general condition of the body, recovery, or death
- To give emergency treatment if necessary

General Instructions

- The pulse may be felt over any large artery that is close to the surface of the body and has a boney structure or other solid surface beneath. Common arteries used for counting the pulse rate are
  - Radial
  - Facial
  - Temporal
  - Dorsalis Pedis
  - Carotid
  - Femoral

- Tibial
- Popliteal

Equipments

- Watch
- Chart and Pen

Procedure

- Keep the patient in a comfortable position
- Hold the wrist firmly, place first three fingers over the artery, press it to make the pulsation distinct.
- Count the pulse for one minute
- Note rhythm, volume and any other abnormalities
- Record your observation

Common Abnormalities in Pulse Rate

- Tachycardia is an abnormally elevated heart rate above 100 beats per minute in adults.
- Bradycardica is a slow rate, below 60 beats per minute in adults.

Rhythm Normally a regular interval occurs between each pulse.

Abnormal rhythm: When there is irregular interval or a missed beat that condition is abnormal rhythm. When dysarrhythmic occurs repetitively, it threatens the hearts ability to provide adequate cardiac output.

Strength: The strength of a pulse reflects two volume of blood ejected against the arterial wall with each heart contraction. Normally the pulse strength remains same. Pulse strength may be graded as strong, weak, thready or bounding. Equality Normally the pulse in one extremity is equal in strength and rate. In some disease condition it may be unequal. Eg. clot formation, injury to blood vessels cervical rib syndrome.

The carotid pulse should never be measured simultaneously because excessive pressure may occlude the blood supply to the brain. Respiration Human survival depends on the ability of oxygen to reach body cells and for CO2 to be removed from the cells.

Respiration is the mechanism the body uses to exchange

gases between the atmosphere and the blood and the blood and the cells. Respiration involves:

- Ventilation
- Diffusion and
- Perfusion

Definition Respiration is the act of breathing. It is made up of one inspiration, one expiration and one pause.

- Ventilation the movement of gases in and out of the lungs. The rate, depth and rhythm of ventilatory movements indicate the quality and efficiency of ventilation.
- Diffusion is the movement of oxygen and CO2 between the alveoli and the red blood cells.
- Perfusion is the distribution of red blood cells to and from the pulmonary capillaries.

Physiological regulation Breathing is generally a passive process. The respiratory centre in the brain stem regulates the involuntary control of respiration. The most important factor in the control of ventilation is the level of CO2 in the blood. An elevation of CO2 in arterial blood causes the respiratory control system in the brain to increase the rate and depth of breathing. The increased ventilatory effort removes excess CO2 during exhalation.

- *Eupnea:* Condition where there is normal rate and depth of Ventilation.
- *Respiratory rate:* Adults normally breath smoothly 12 to 20 times a minute.

Characters of respiration

- *Respiratory rate:* the nurse observe a full inspiration and expiration when counting ventilation or respiration rate.
- Ventilatory depth is the degree of excursion or movement in the chest wall. Ventilatory movements may be deep, normal or shallow.
  - Deep respiration involves a full expansion of the lungs with full exhalation.
  - Shallow respiration: is present when only a small

quantity of air passes through the lungs and ventilatory movement is difficult to see.

- *Ventilatory rhythm:* With normal breathing, a regular interval occurs after each respiratory cycle. Respiration is regular or irregular in rhythm.

Factors Which Regulate Respiration

- Respiratory centre in the medulla
- Nerve fibres of the autonomic nervous system.
- Chemical composition of blood.

What to Note When Taking Respiration

- Rate and depth
- Movement and expansion of chest and abdomen.
- Rhythm.
- Whether quiet or noisy.
- Comfort of the patient, whether breathing is done unconsciously or with effort.

Procedure:

- Keep the patient in a relaxed and comfortable position.
- Try to count the respirations without the patient knowing that you are watching him or he may change the rate of respiration.
- Keep the fingers on the patient' s wrist, as if for counting pulse and watch the rise and fall of the chest and abdomen or if the patient is sitting watch the movements of the shoulders.
- Chart the rate and record any abnormalities.

Frequency of Monitoring Respiration

- Twice a day for all patients.
- Every four hours for postoperative patients.
- Every 30 minutes for immediate postoperative patients.
- Every 15 minutes for critically ill patients.

Alteration in (Abnormal) Breathing Patterns

- *Brady pnea:* The respiratory is abnormally slow (less

than 12 breaths per minute) Occurs in coma due to cerebral haemmorrhage or large doses of sedatives,

- *Tachy pnea:* The respiratory rate is abnormally rapid (greater than 20 breaths per minute)
- *Apnea:* Respirations cease for several seconds.
- *Respiratory arrest:* Persistant cessation of respiration.
- *Hyper Ventilation:* Rate and depth of respirations increase.
- *Hypoventilation:* Rate is abnormally low and depth is shallow. Shallow respiration occurs in diseases of the lung such as pneumonia and pleurisy.
- *Sighing or air hunger:* Indicates a need for more oxygen. Occurs in severe haemorrhage diabetic coma or due to stimulation of respiratory centre by excess of acid.
- *Wheezing:* Sound made during expiration may be due to obstruction in the lower respiratory tract as in the case of asthma.
- *Stertorous breathing:* Noisy snoring inspiration occurs in unconscious patients which may be due to the tongue slipping back. Peculiar hissing respiraton occurs in uraemic coma.
- *Stridor:* It is noisy inspiration due to the obstruction of upper respiratory tract. This noise may be harsh, grating or whistling sound.
- *Orthopnea:* Inability to breath easily unless in an upright position.
- *Dyspnoea:* Difficult breathing. If it is during inspiration it is due to laryngeal obstruction; if it is during expiration it is due to Asthma.
- *Cheyne stokes or periodic breathing:* Alternative periods of hyperponea, occuring in a rhythmical cycle. It is important to note this phenomenon as this is a serious sign.
- *Asphyxia:* Occurs due to lack of oxygen supplied to the cells.

  This is found in drowning patients of persons who have inhaled poisonous gases (coal gas).

BLOOD PRESSURE

Blood Pressure (BP) is the lateral force on the walls of artery by the pulsing blood under pressure from the heart. The heart' s contraction forces blood under high pressure into the aorta. The peak of maximum pressure when ejection occurs is the systolic blood pressure.

When the ventricles relax, the blood remaining in the arteries exerts a minimum a diastolic pressure. Diastolic pressure is the minimal pressure exerted against the arterial walls at all times.

The standard unit for measuring blood pressure is millimeters of mercury (mmHg). The BP is recorded with the systolic reading before diastolic. Eg. 120 / 80 mmHg. 120 is systolic pressure 80 is diastolic pressure The difference between systolic and diastolic pressure is the pulse pressure.

PHYSIOLOGY OF BP

BP reflects inter relationship of cardiac output, peripheral vascular resistance.

- Cardiac output is the volume of blood pumped by the heart (stroke volume) during one minute.
- Cardiac output = Heart rate x stroke volume
- The BP depends on the cardiac output and peripheral vascular resistance (R).
- BP = Cardiac output x R
- Peripheral vascular resistance is the resistance to blood flow determined by the vascular wall and diameter of blood vessels when the diameter is less, the vascular resistance to blood flow is increased.
- Blood volume the volume of blood circulating with in vascular system, affects BP. For adults, normal circulating blood volume is 5000 ml. If volume increases, BP elevates.
  Eg. rapid uncontrolled intravenous fluid. When circulating volume falls, blood pressure falls. Eg. haemorrhage, dehydration.
- *Elasticity*: Normally the arterical walls are elastic and easily distensible. Contain diseases such as

arteriosclerosis, lose their elasticity and cannot stretch wall. When the blood is forced into blood vessels, due to the rigid blood walls, the systolic pressure rises.

Factors Influencing Variations in BP

- *Age:* Normal BP levels vary through out life larger children have higher BP than smaller children of same age.
- *Stress:* Anxiety, fear pain and emotional stress result in increase in heart rate resulting in increasing in BP.
- *Race:* Certain race are more prone for high BP. Genetically and environmentally.
- *Medication:* Some medications can affect BP directly or indirectly.
- *Diurnal variation:* BP levels vary over the course of a day. BP is lowest in the early morning, gradually arises during morning and afternoon and peaks in evening.
- *Gender:* After puberty males tend to have higher BP. After, menopause, women tend to have high BP. BP is measured by sphygmomanometer.

Variation in BP

- Hypertension: Elevated or high blood pressure is known as hyper tension. Hyper tension is a major factor causing deaths from strokes and myocardial infarction (Heart arrest)

Causes of Hypertension

- Family history of Hypertension.
- Obesity
- Cigarette smoking,
- Aalcohol consumption,
- High blood cholesterol level,
- Continued exposure to stress,
- Old age.

Treatment

- Early diagnosis,
- Long-term follow up care and therapy.

Hypotension: When the systolic pressure falls to 90 mm Hg or below, that condition is known as hypo tension.

Causes of Hypotension

- Dilatation of the arteries.
- Loss of blood, Due to haemorrhage.
- Failure of heart muscle to pump adequately (Heart attack)

Signs Symptoms of Hypotension

- Pallor,
- Skin mottling,
- Cold and clammey
- Increased heart rate.
- Decreased urine output.

Monitoring BP Purposes

- To aid in the diagnosis of the patient' s condition
- To guide in his treatment.
- To evaluate the patient' s progress.

General Instructions

- See that the patient is relaxed and is a comfortable position.
- Help to take blood pressure for patients with the following conditions.
  - New patients.
  - Pre and post operative patients.
  - Antenatal and post natal patients.
  - Patients with shock and haemorrhage.
  - Patients with cardiac conditions and hypertension
  - Patients with neurological disorders.
- Record pulse along with blood pressure.
- Blood pressure is taken at the same arm, same time, same posture daily.

Equipments

- Sphygmomanometer.

- Stethescope.
- Pen.

Guidelines

- The sphygmomanometers generally used in clinical setting are mercury type. And aneroid type. The mercury type sphygmomanometers are more reliable than the aneroid type sphygmoma-nometers. The aneroid sphygmomanometers gives blood pressure reading on dial indicator.
- Systolic pressure is increased in pressure induced by systolic contraction and diastolic pressure is decrease in pressure induced by diastolic relaxation of the left ventricle of heart.
- Never take blood pressure when the patient is excited, exhausted and just after exercise, smoking or meals.
- Allow the patient to rest for five minutes before taking blood pressure.
- Do not use the extremity that is injured, diseased, paralysed, receiving intravenous infusion or when a female patient is with radical mastectomy on the same side.
- When the arm cannot be used to measure the blood pressure, the thigh can be used being a good alternative site.
- Always take the blood pressure reading on the same side and in the same position to maintain consistency.
- Place the site (arm or leg) about the level of heart while taking blood pressure.
- The apparatus should be in working order. The cuff should be of appropriate size (12-14 cm for arm and 18- 20 cm for thigh) and deflated before wrapping around the patient' s site.
- While taking blood pressure, certain sounds are heard in sequence. These are called as Korotkoff sounds and are described as under.
  - TappingThe faint clear sounds that gradually become louder, the first tapping sound may be

followed by an absence of sound (auscultatory gap)and indicates systolic pressure reading.
- Murmuring The low swishing sounds that increase with cuff deflation.
- Knocking The crisp, clear sounds that occur with each heart beat.
- Muffling Abrupt change of sound indicates first diastolic pressure reading.
- No sounds The sound disappears and indicates second diastolic pressure reading.

- When deflating the cuff to take the readings, deflate the cuff to 0. Do not stop in between and start inflating again as this gives a false reading.
- Note the variations in blood pressure.

Procedure

- Explain the procedure to patient. See patient is relaxed and is in a comfortable position. Support the arm.
- Expose the arm and keep it extended.
- Apply the end of the cuff with the rubber bag over the brachial artery two inches above the elbow.
- Apply the end of the cuff smoothly and snugly around the upper arm. Tuck the end neatly.
- Place the Sphygmomanometer in position.
- Stay with the patient until the procedure is over.
- Remove the cuff from the patient' s arm, roll neatly and replace in the box. See patient is comfortable.
- The reading is recorded in the chart.
- Systolic pressure is always written over the diastolic pressure Eg.120/80mm/Hg.

Chapter 8

Modes of Communication

Communication is the basic element of human interaction that allows people to establish, maintain and improve contacts with other. Communication is defined as a process of exchange of thought or an idea from one individual to another individual through verbal language or gesture.

Communication refers to nonverbal and verbal behaviour within a social context and includes all symbols and clues used by people to give and receive meaning. Communication is an important component of nursing practice. To communicate effectively with patients, nurses must develop skilled communication techniques.

Process of Communication

The basic elements of communication are:

- The referent,
- The sender,
- The message,
- The channels,
- The receiver,
- Environment,
- Feedback,

The Communication Process

- The Sender is the person who initiates the interpersonal communication.
- The message is the information sent by the sender.
- Channels are means of conveying, messages.
- Receiver is the person to whom the messages is sent.

- The environment is the physical and emotional atmosphere present at the time of interaction.
- Feedback is the return message of the receiver to the sender.
- Referent may be an object, emotion or experience that motivates one person to communicate with another.

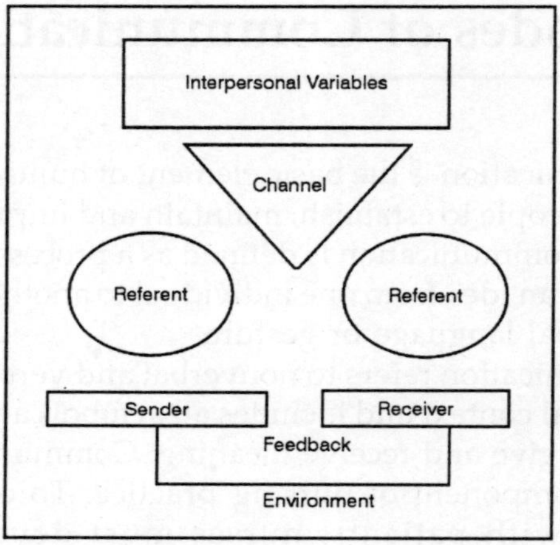

Modes of Communication

- Verbal Communication involves the spoken or written word. Clear messages require using effective verbal communication techniques.
- Nonverbal Communication is the exchange of a message without using words.

Level of Communication

- Interpersonal Communication is the interaction between two people or in a small group.
- Public Communication is the interaction with large groups of people.
- Interpersonal Communication is the way people consider their thoughts internally so that they can express themselves appropriately to others.

Characteristics of Effective Communication

- Maintaining silence.

- Listening attentively.
- Willingness to hear a message.
- Asking related questions.
- Paraphrasing or restating the message.
- Focusing on a specific topic.
- Summarizing (or) concise review of main ideas at the end.

Factors that Influence Communication

- Perceptions of individuals.
- Values.
- Development stage.
- Space.
- Gender.
- Emotions.
- Socio-cultural background..
- Knowledge.
- Roles and relationships. 10) Environmental setting.

Factors Inhibiting Effective Communication

- Giving an opinion.
- Offering false assurance.
- Being defensive.
- Showing approval or disapproval.
- Asking why.
- Changing the subject inappropriately.
- Forming communication barriers by inadvertently saying something that blocks the communication process.

THERAPEUTIC COMMUNICATION (OR) NURSE - PATIENT RELATIONSHIP

Without knowing the patient' s needs, a nurse is unable to effectively diagnose, response to illness and initiate actions. Through therapeutic.

Relationship, the nurse develops a working, functional relationship with patients and fulfil purpose of nursing process.

Social Interaction

Social interaction is the first attempt at communicating with a patient. The messages conveyed are usually superficial. A social interaction at the beginning of conversation is necessary to establish a close relationship of trust. (eg) The nurse might greet a client by saying "Good morning, Mrs. Rani" A skillful nurse maintains a congenial and warm style of communicating to elicit a patient' s trust. The nurse' s goal is to help the clients to feel comfortable in sharing attitudes and feelings.

Developing a Helping Relationship

- Nurse-patient relationship is the learning experience whereby two people interact to face an immediate health problem, to share, if possible in resolving it and to discover ways to adapt to the situation. The nurse uses interpersonal communication skills to develop a relationship that will lead to understanding the patient as a total person. The relationship in therapeutic, promotes positive change and growth.

Dimension of Helping Relationship

- Trust is the assured belief that other individuals are capable of assisting in times of distress. Trust fosters open, therapeutic communication. To foster trust, the nurse acts consistently, reliably and competently. Honesty also builds trust.
- Empathy is the ability to understand and accept the life of another person and to accurately perceive feeling. The nurses communicates an understanding of the client' s expressions.
- Caring is the foundation of nursing as a human science. Caring attitudes involves.
  - Attention to or concern for the patient.
  - Responsibility for the patient and
  - Regard, fondness or attachment to a patient. A nurse shows caring by accepting patients for themselves and respecting them as individuals.

Autonomy and Mutuality

Autonomy refers to ability to be self-directed. Mutuality involves sharing with another. The nurse and patient work as a team. Nurse offers patients opportunity to make decision and works with the patient to achieve and maintain an optimal level of wellness. Communicating with Children involves sitting at eye level, using simple direct language and incorporating play into discussion.

Communication with older adult patients with sensory losses require communication techniques that maximize existing sensory and motor function. Communication is one of the most important skill for a nurse. Through communication a nurse establishes a relationship with patients and families to help them acquire healthy behaviour.

COMMUNICATION IN HEALTH EDUCATION

Health education mainly depends upon good communication. The purpose of communication is to transmit information from one person or group of people to another person or group, with a view to bringing about desirable behavioural change. In communication, ideas must travel between the sender and the receiver that is between the speaker and listener or writer and reader. In effective communication the receiver must understand the message correctly.

Need for Communication

- To get along with people
- To understand people (patients, team workers, friends, etc) and, in turn, to be understood.
- To gain their confidence and respect, especially patients and community, and to be respected.

The key Elements in the Communication Process Are

- Communicator or sender, He is the originator of the message, his objectives must be clearly stated. In health education the nurse is the originator of the message.

- Message, It should be carefully chosen, Valid, useful and understandable. It must be arranged in proper sequence (order)
- Audience. They are the receives or consumers of the message and they respond to the message.
- Channels of communication. The media through which the message is sent.

Barriers to Communication

- Physical - The receiver may have some problem or handicaps for example he may not be able to listen.
- Psychological - Emotional disturbances, worry, anxiety. Environmental noise, congestion, invisibility etc.
- Cultural - strong beliefs, customs, attitudes, religious sentiments, illiteracy etc.

Key to Effective Communication

Just as keys are used to open strong locks to reveal what is inside, effective communication will help to overcome most of the barriers in communication. First of all we must understand our own ideas and beliefs before we talk to others. Plan your communication.

You must be known what you want to say and how to say it and to whom to say it. Think before you talk, use the right word in the right place, to the right person, at the right time and in the right manner.

People not only hear what you say but how you say it and observe your facial expressions, voice, actions and other clues that convey the real message. Once the message is sent and received allow for a feedback, that is giving a change for the receiver to let you know what they have understood. Be a good listener and allow the receiver to talk and to convey his ideas and feelings. It is important in the patient nurse relationship to help the patient tell his problems and feelings, which will help proper diagnosis and treatment.

Make use of your five senses - touch, taste, smell, hearing and sight for clauses in the receiver. Observe with the intent to understand and report to a senior nurse when necessary. Do not interrupt when others are talking. Try to understand just as you would like to be understood. As important function of the nurse is to get to know the sick and the well in need of help, effective communication will be helpful to a large extent.

Education

Education is a process of learning and experience, through which knowledge is acquired and attitudes are developed to result in intelligent and skillful behaviour. Teaching is the art of inducting and helping people to learn. The teacher only induces and helps, but the actual knowledge must be acquired by the effort of the learner himself.

- What is learning? Learning is doing.
- Under what conditions do we learn better?
  - When do we need to learn?
  - When are we known of what our goals or aims?
  - When do we learn in a practicals?
  - At what time do we reward and punish?
  - When do we connect that is being learned with something we already knew or familiar with.
  - When do our learning signifies the personal meaning ?
  - When do we learn through emotional experiences?
  - When do we know to apply our knowledge and skills that are already learnt?
- What are some ways in which we can help people to learn?
  - We should make our points clear.
  - Whenever possible, we should demonstrate what we want people to learn.
  - We should make the group feel secured(friendly and at ease).
  - We should encourage free discussion among people.
- What are causes of non-learning?
  - Use of poor teaching method.

- Poor health of the learner.
- Frustration of the learner because his needs have not been met.
- Worries of the learners.
- Bad home and work conditions.
- Standards too high for learned to understand.
- Use of difficult instead of simple teaching methods.
- Helping the learner so much that he does not learn to help himself. Health is only one aspect of human welfare and does not exist in isolation. It is closely lined with others such as housing, economy, security, agricultural property and so on. For prevention of disease and promotion of health, health education is one of the most important functions of the health team.

  The nurse should know some of the common methods of health teaching so that she can select the most suitable methods for individual and group teaching. Some of these methods that the nurse uses will depend on the groups educational background and their experience with the situations and their experience of work.

- Why should we use health education materials or media? We use materials
  - To provide information
  - To encourage change in attitudes
  - To stimulate change in behaviour.
- What should we look for when selecting materials for use in health education?
  - The contents should be scientifically accurate.
  - They should be understood by the people.
  - The material should be brief and simple.
  - The material should be attractive.
  - The material should be up to date and timely.
  - It should have a central theme or idea.
  - It should suggest action to be followed by the people.

Chapter 9

First aid and Emergencies

First aid was being practical from ancient times. It was the famous surgeon who was the first to conceive the idea of first aid. He was General Esmarch (1823-1908). In 1877 St John Ambulance Association of England was formed in 1920, The Red Cross society of India was established with more than 400 branches all over India.

DEFINITIONS MEDICAL AID

Refers to treatment by a doctor either on the sport at home or in the hospital First Aid is the immediate and temporary care given to an injured or sick person until the services of a qualified doctor aré obtained with such material as may be available.

The first aid is not an end by itself. It indicates that the person is in need of a secondary aid. First aid is based on the knowledge of biology, medicine and surgery. It can be a life saving skill.

First aider: The person who renders emergency service on the spot until the medical aid is obtained.

A sound knowledge based on first aid enables a nurse to give skilled services during accidents and sudden illness to preserve life promote recovery and prevent injury or illness being aggravated until the medical aid has been obtained.
Objectives

- To save life
- Adverse effects of injury are controlled.
- To ease the Pain-to reduce Pain.
- To avoid further injury.

- Prepare for medical treatment
- To assist the doctor.

Scope of First Aid

- Diagnosis: Observation and information elicited will enable for diagnosis.
- Treatment: The nurse (nurse) decides on the character and extends of the treatment and applies the most suitable treatment until the doctor' s help is available.

Basic Principles and Rules of First aid

- Obtain a correct detailed history
- Observe and examine thoroughly and note every symptom.
- Treat the casualty until the details arrives or patient is shifted to the near by hospital.
- If the accident is at home- call neighbour, if the accident is at the public place -call police
- Keep phone numbers of doctor, police control room.

Golden Rules

- Be calm and quick, be methodical and find out all major injuries.
- In stoppage of breathing, start artificial respiration.
- Try to stop bleeding.
- Prevent shock if present and shift to near by hospital
- Keep the patient warm. Do not move unnecessarily
- Do only what is necessary.
- Reassure the casualty
- Avoid crowd.
- Allow fresh air
- Quickest means of transport at emergency
- For serious accident inform police.

ACCIDGENTS

An accident is an event, which happens unexpectedly. The extent of the injury depends on various factors. The accidents, which are most likely to come across, are as follows.

- Wounds
- Sprains and dislocations

- Fractures (broken bones)
- Burns and scalds. Some times there may be a history given that the patient has received an injury to the head or some other part of the body but there is no visible injury. However in these cases the patient may be unconscious, may show signs of shock or may complain of pain. In all such cases you transfer the patient to the Health Centre immediately. As you are a nurse and the aim of your assistance is as follows.
- To prevent immediate danger of death.
- Give artificial respiration.
- Guard against shock or treat for shock.
- Do not remove clothing unnecessarily.
- Reassure the patient and relieve pain.
- Arrange for removal of the patient to the nearest Hospital

Wounds

A wound is a tear or break in the skin following an accident. The deeper the wound the more likely it is to bleed and to get infected as it can' t be properly cleaned. You must stop the bleeding and, as far as possible, prevent infection from occurring.

Types of Wounds

- Abrasion: this is usually a superficial wound with peeling of skin.
- Cut, eg. by a knife or other sharp cutting instrument: This is usually accompanied by profuse bleeding and the deeper structures may also be cut.
- Torn, eg, by barbed wire or by a blunt instrument: The edges of the wound are irregular and there is bruising.
- Punctured, eg,. by a knife, nail or bullet: This wound is small but deep so that important organs may be damaged.

Treatment

- Make the patient sit or lie down.
- Handle the injured part gently.

- Wash the wound with clean water and soap. Always clean away form the wound.
- Remove as much dirt or foreign matter as possible.
- Wash the wound with antiseptic lotion.
- Stop any bleeding by using direct pressure or by applying a tourniquet.
- Apply antiseptic solutions (dettol) and dust wound with sulphonamide powder.
- If the wound is gaping, apply strips of adhesive plaster to bring the edges together.
- Apply a clean dressing and bandage. 10) If necessary treat for shock. 1
- Give pain reliever, if policy permits. 1
- Support the arm in a sling when necessary.

You must Always Refer the Patient to the Hospital in the Following Cases

- If the wound is large and needs stitching
- If there is severe bleeding
- If there is shock or the patient is unconscious.
- If there is a foreign body embedded in the wound.
- In all deep wounds of the chest and abdomen.

Haemorrhage

Bleeding or loss of blood accompanies an accident in which a wound, a fracture or damage to organs occurs. If there is oozing or a steady flow of blood, it can usually be controlled by direct pressure on the wound. If however, bleeding is severe and is coming out in spirts, a tourniquet will be needed to control bleeding. A narrow fold triangular bandage, a handkerchief, a necktie, a broad belt or any other piece of material of sufficient length can be used as an improvised tourniquet. The method described here refers to the use of an improvised tourniquet.

- Fold the triangular bandage of handkerchief to a width of 5 cm
- Apply it on clothing at the level of the middle of the upper or lower limb

- Tie the free ends of the bandage in a hal-knot on the outer side of the limb.
- Place a pencil, piece of wood, spoon etc., on the halfknot
- Complete the knot to hold the pencil in position
- Twist the pencil gradually so as to tighten the bandage until the bleeding stops.
- Use a second bandage tied around the limb to keep the pencil in the tightened up position
- Leave the tourniquet in place, but loosen it gently every 15 minutes.
- If the bleeding has stopped, leave he tourniquet in place but do not tighten up again
- If the bleeding starts again, tighten the tourniquet and repeat steps vi, vii, viii
- Go with the patient to the hospital, if possible so the you can control the bleeding
- Attach a label or any piece of paper to the patient' s shirt showing the time when the tourniquet was applied.

Note: A tourniquet is a very useful appliance to use in the presence of open fractures of a limb.

Control of Bleeding From the Nose

Nosebleeds are fairly common and are due to rupture of small vessels in the walls of the nostrils. If the bleeding does not stop refer the patient to the medical aid.

Electric Shock

An electric shock is caused by a person touching a live electric wire. The signs of electric shock are as follows.

- The patient is unconscious.
- The patient is in contact with a source of electricity. When you see a person who has an electric shock you must act promptly in order to save his life. Proceed as follows:
- Whenever possible shut off the current.
- Free the person from the source of electricity by using

a piece of wood, paper or rubber to push or pull him away.

- If there is cessation of breath, give mouth-to mouth respiration immediately. (refer CPR). Mouth to mouth respiration should be continued for a long time, and certainly for as long as the respiration is restored.
- After the patient has recovered, examine the skin for the presence of any burns and refer to the person for further treatment.
- Educate the community on how to avoid electric shock by talking on the following points. o Ensure that all electric points are safe and that there are no exposed live wires.
  - Prevent children from playing with electric switches and sockets.
  - Prevent children from climbing up electric poles.

Heat Stroke

Heat stroke results from exposure to excessive heat and sun and may occur during the hot summer months. It is more likely to occur in those who have been drinking alcohol and those who are weak. The early signs and symptoms of heat stroke are as follows:

- High temperature (up to 42 C)
- Headache
- Dizziness
- Nausea and vomiting
- Cramps in the limbs
- Dry flushed, hot skin The patient may become unconscious later on.

When this happens he usually dies. When you see a patient with heatstroke proceed as follows.

- Put him in the shade in the coolest and most cold clothes.
- Undress him completely
- Cover the head and back of the neck with a turban or towel when exposed to the sun for long periods.

- If conscious provide cool water.

Sprains, Dislocations and Fractures

These occur when a joint is twisted by tripping or falling, or by a sudden wrench. In a sprain the joint is not displaced, while in a dislocation part of the joint is displaced.

Fractures

A fracture is a broken bone, it may be cracked, broken into two or more pieces. Further fractures may be classified:

- Closed: there is no wound leading down to the bone and there is no bone protruding through the skin
- Open: there is a wound reaching form the skin right down to the broken bone, or the broken bone may protrude through the wound You must remember the following rules when dealing with a fracture:
- All fractures should be given first aid treatment and sent to the hospital.
- Interfere as little as possible with a fracture and do only what is absolutely necessary to prepare the patient for the transfer to the hospital.
- Immobilize the fractured part.

Signs and Symptoms

- History of a fall or a fit.
- Pain at the site or near the site of fracture
- Inability to move the fractured limb
- Swelling at the site of fracture
- Fracture may be felt
- Movement at the place where there should be no movement
- Broken end of bone seen protruding under the skin.

Treatment

- Place the patient in a comfortable position with the injured part well supported
- Do not remove clothing
- Immobilize the injured part by using a splint and bandages

- Always immobilize the joint above and below the fracture site
- Treat for shock, but do not give any drink, as the patient may have to have an anaesthesia for setting the fracture on arrival to the hospital.
- Inform the medical aid If the fracture is an open one, in addition to the six steps mentioned, carry out the following
- Cut away
- Remove the clothing over the wound and
- Cover it with a clean dry dressing.
- Stop any bleeding by applying a pad and bandage.
- If the bleeding is severe and comes out in spurts
- Apply a tourniquet.

Burns and Scalds

Burns are caused by dry heat such as fire, explosion of pressure stoves, petrol burns, hot metals and electrocution. Corrosive chemicals such as strong acid from batteries of cars also cause burns. Scalds produce the same type of injury as burns and are caused by wet heat such as boiling water, steam, hot oil or ghee and tar. The treatment of burns and scalds will depend on whether the skin is intact or only partially destroyed or whether it is completely destroyed.

Bites and Stings Snake Bite

Snake bite results in punctured wounds caused by the fangs of a snake. The wounds by themselves are minor ones, you should always treat the bite as poisonous.

Dog Bite

In India where rabies is prevalent, if a person by a bitten by a stray Dog the injury should be taken seriously. Wounds from dog bite are infected because dirt and germs are introduced into the wound from the teeth of the dog.

Scorpion Sting

The person stung by a scorpion, usually a child, complains

of severe pain at the site of the sting and signs of shock. A scorpion sting is poisonous, and if the child is small and physically weak the sting may produce serious results.

Drowning

Drowning occurs when the person has inhaled the water into the lungs. The lungs become full of water instead of air. If a person who has drowned is brought, the nurse should proceed the first aid as follows.

- Turn the patient face down with the head turned to one side and the arms stretched out. If a slope exists, the head must be placed downwards.
- Place your hand around the patient' s abdomen and raise the body to encourage the water to run out of the lungs.
- Clear the mouth of weeds or any other material obstructing air entity, and of false teeth if any. Loosen the clothing around the neck and waist.
- Apply artificial respiration using the method mentioned in CPR.
- Do not stop until the breathing has been reestablished for at least a quarter of an hour.
- After recovery do not let the patient sit up. Transfer him/her lying on a stretcher to the nearest hospital as soon as possible.

POISONING

Substances, when taken into the body in fairly large quantities, can be dangerous to health or can cause death, are called poisons.

Types of Poisons

Swallowed Poisons

Acids, alkaline, disinfectant, tablets for sleeping, tranquilizers and pain killing drugs. Alcoholic drink taken in large quantities Inhaled poisons.

Fumes and gases from explosions and fires cause choking,

difficulty in breathing and death. Injected poisons Poisons get into the body through injections.

First Aid in Poisoning

- Poisoning is a serious matter
- Patient must be removed to a hospital or a doctor
- Preserve packets or bottles, which you suspect contained the poison

If the Victim is Unconscious

Do not induce Vomiting

- Make the causality lie on his back or on a hard flat bed without any pillow and turn the head to one side.
- If breathing is very slow or stopped, start artificial respiration and keep it up, till the doctor comes/ respiration gets restored.

If the Victim is Conscious

- Aid vomiting by tickling the back of the throat 2. Make him drink tepid water mixed with two tablespoons of common salt for a tumbler of water 3. If it is a corrosive poison do not induce vomiting Signs of corrosive poisons Lips, mouth, and skin show grey, white or yellow patches.

Management

1 The poison must be diluted by giving large quantities of cold water. This will dilute the irritant and delay absorption. 2. Milk, egg beaten are given for the above purpose

Foreign Bodies Eye

Foreign bodies such as insects and pieces of grit often enter the eye and may be quite difficult to discover. They produce feeling of discomfort and grittiness, which is accompanied by redness, congestion and watering. These symptoms and signs are similar to those caused by disease. Therefore after a careful search, if the nurse fails to discover a foreign body she must at once refer the patient to a doctor.

Ear

- If it is an insect, fill the ear with glycerine or cocanut, or mustard oil or warm salt water.
- The insect will float up and can be removed easily.
- If there is nothing floating up, leave it alone. Do not meddle.
- Never pour the water and irrigate the ear since this may cause damage to the ear drum. For blockage due to hardened blocks take to him to the doctor.

Nose

- Children often insert foreign bodies such as buttons, pencil and beads into the nose.
- The child herself calls attention.
- Unless it is obviously easy to remove the foreign body, the nurse should not try to remove.
- The child should be warned not to inhale through her nose because this provokes the danger of drawing the foreign body further upwards.
- Advice mouth breathing until removing the foreign body. Refer the child to the doctor.

Throat

Some small objects like safety pin, irregular objects, fish bone or prawn get lodged or obstruct the throat. The nurse should refer the victim to the doctor

Stomach

Smooth object like buttons, coins, nuts, safety pin etc are swallowed. The nurse should refer the patient to the doctor.

CARDIOPULMONARY EMERGENCIES

CARDIAC EMERGENCY (CPR)

First aid for cardiopulmonary arrest Establish unresponsiveness

- When you first discover the victim, look at him closely. Shake him gently by the shoulders and shout "Are you okay?". This "shaking and shouting" will establish whether or not he is unconscious.
- Observe A.B.C. of resuscitation - A = Airway, B = Breathing, C = Circulation.

Open the airway

Open the victim's airway. The most common cause of airway obstruction in an unconscious person is the tongue, which has relaxed and fallen into the airway. Because the tongue is attached to the lower jaw, moving the lower jaw forward will lift the tongue away from the back of the throat, opening the airway. You can use three methods to open the airway: the preferred head-tilt/chin-lift, the head-tilt/neck-lift, or the jaw thrust without head-tilt.

To use the head-tilt/chin-lift method, place your hands that is closest to the victim's head on his forehead and tilt his head slightly. Place the fingertips of your other hand under his lower jaw on the bony part near the chin. Gently lift the chin up, taking care not to close his mouth.

To use the head-tilt/neck-lift method, place the palm of your hand that is closest to the victim' s head on his forehead and your other hand under his neck. Place the hand lifting his neck close to the back of his head to minimize cervical-spine extension. Then gently press back on his forehead while lifting up and supporting his neck. Use the jaw-thrust without head-tilt method if you suspect the victim has a neck or spine injury. Kneel at the victim' s head, facing his feet. Place your thumbs on his mandible near the corners of his mouth, pointing your thumbs toward his feet.

Then position the tips of your index fingers at the angles of his jaw. Push your thumbs down while you lift upward with the tips of your index fingers. This action should open the victim' s airway. Once you have opened the victim's airway see if this action alone has restored his breathing. Put your ear over his mouth and nose while you look forward his chest and abdomen. Listen for any air movement and look to see if his chest or abdomen is moving up and down. Feel with your chest for any flow of air. If the victim has started to breathe, maintain his airway until help arrives.

- If the victim hasn't started to breathe, close his nostrils with the thumb and index finger of your hand on his forehead.
- Open your mouth wide and place it over the victim' s mouth, sealing it tightly so that no air can escape.
- When you use the jaw-thrust method to open the airway, you must tuck your cheek under his nostrils.
- Deliver four quick breaths
  - Don' t allow the victim to exhale between these breaths.
  - These four breaths maintain positive pressure in the airway.

Even if the victim has stopped breathing for only for a short time, some of his lungs' alveoli may have collapsed. Positive pressure helps reinflate them. When you see the victim' s chest rise, then fall (after your fourth breath), you will know that air is entering and escaping his lungs. If the victim wears dentures, keeping them in place will usually make ventilation easier. But if they are slipping, remove them.

RESTORE CIRCULATION

- Now locate the victim's carotid pulse. To do so, keep your hand on his forehead to maintain the head-tilt position. Use your other hand to find the carotid artery on the side closest to you, in the groove beside the larynx. Use your index and middle fingers to gently palpate the artery for 5 to 10 seconds.
- If you find a pulse, don't give cardiac compressions but do ventilate the patient at a rate of one breath every seconds (12 breaths a minute).
- Continue to check his pulse after every 12 breaths. If you find no pulse, prepare to begin cardiac compression. Position yourself close to the victim' s side, with your knees apart. This position gives you a broad base of support.

- Use the fingers of your hand that' s closest to the victim' s feet to lower margin of his rib cage and trace the margin to the notch where the ribs meet the sternum.
- Next, place your middle finger on the notch.
- Place your index finger of the same hand next to your middle finger. Then place the heel of your other hand next to your index finger on the long axis of the sternum, as shown.
- This is the correct position for cardiac compression. If your hands are placed incorrectly, you may lacerate the victim' s liver or fracture a rib.
- Place the hand you used to locate the notch over the heel of your other hand. Interlock or extend your fingers to keep them off the victim' s ribs and to maintain vertical pressure through the heel of the hand touching the sternum.
- Align your shoulders over your hands, keeping your elbows straight. Keeping your fingers off the ribs and your shoulders aligned ensures that you will compress downward, not laterally. Lateral compressions won' t deliver sufficient pressure. 10) Using the weight of your upper body, compress downward about 1.1/2 to 2 inches (3 to 5 cm), concentrating the pressure through the heels of your hands.
- Don' t deliver bouncing compressions because they are less effective and could injure the victim. Then relax the pressure completely to let the victim' s heart fill with blood.
- Don' t remove your hands from his chest when you relax, or you will lose your hand position.
- If you are the only rescuer, time your compressions at a rate of 80 a minute. Count, "One and two and three and four and five and ..." up to the count of fifteen.
- Then deliver two quick breaths without allowing the victim to exhale between them. (Actually, you will be delivering 60 compressions a minute, with the delay to ventilate the victim).

- Perform CPR for 1 minute, check the victim' s pulse, then quickly telephone for help if none has arrived. Return quickly and resume CPR. If there is no phone available, continue CPR.
- If a second rescuer arrives, ask her to call or go for help if you have not been able to do so. Then she can help you resuscitate the victim.
(Of course, she must be trained in CPR if she is going to assist you).
- Have the second rescuer get on the opposite side of the victim' s airway, across from you. As she opens the victim' s airway and tries to locate the carotid pulse, you continue giving compressions.
- If your compressions are strong enough, she should feel a pulse. When the second rescuer signal that she has found the pulse you are generating, stop your compressions for 5 seconds so she can see if the victim' s heart is beating on its own.
- If she can' t feel a spontaneous pulse, she should deliver one breathe. You can then resume compressions (approximately 60 per minute), while the second rescuer delivers a full breath on the upstroke of every fifth compression.
- To assure that you work as a team, count out loud: "One thousand one, one thousand two, one thousand three, one thousand four, one thousand five, one thousand..." and so on. Have the second rescuer check for the victim' s pulse every few minutes.
- When you feel tired, tell the second rescuer you want to switch positions. To alert her, say: "Switch, one thousand, two, one thousand, five, one thousand". When you finish this count, the second rescuer should be delivering a full breath as you a move toward the victim' s head.
- When you get to his head, open his airway and assess his carotid pulse for 5 seconds. The second rescuer should get into position for cardiac compression.
- If you can' t feel a pulse, deliver one breath and tell

the second rescuer to start the compressions. If you do find a pulse but the victim is not breathing, tell the second rescuer not to give any compression.

- Continue giving the victim mouth-mouth ventilation and check his pulse every few minutes, in case his heart stops again.

Cardiopulmonary resuscitation for small children and infants is similar to that for adults.

- Generally, a child younger than a year is considered an infant, and one between 1 and 8 years old is considered a small child.
- Use adult CPR techniques for children older than 8 years. In an emergency, of course, you are not going to delay CPR until you determine the child' s age. Instead, consider his body size relation to the size of your hand.
- For example, if he looks too small to use both hands for cardiac compression, use the heel of one hand. If he is too small for that, use two or three fingers.

CPR FOR SMALL CHILDREN

- Use the head-tilt/neck-lift (as shown) or head-tilt/chinlift method to open the airway. You may need to use two or three fingers instead of your whole hand to lift the child' s neck if it is very small.
- If you use the head-tilt/chin-lift method, be careful not to close the child' s mouth when you lift his chin. Also, be sure your fingers are not pressing on the soft tissue under his chin, which may cause edema and subsequent airway obstruction.
- If the child' s face is large enough, maintain a tight seal by pinching his nostrils (as shown) and placing your mouth over his.
- If he has a small face, place your mouth over his mouth and nose. When ventilating, give only enough air to make the child' s chest rise.
- Try to palpate the child' s carotid pulse. If you find a pulse, do not give cardiac compression but do ventilate the child at a rate of one breath every 4 seconds.

- If you can' t locate a pulse, find the proper location for compression.

Use the same Technique you Would for an Adult.

- Then compress about 1 to 1.1/2 inches (2.5 to 3.8 cm), using the heel of one hand (as shown).
- Give 80 compressions a minute, with a breath after every fifth compression. Your count should be: "One and two and three and four and five and one..." and so on.
- This rate and ratio are the same if you have a second rescuer helping you, but the second rescuer should ventilate on the upstroke of the fifth compression.

CPR for Infants

- When you tilt an infant' s head, you will lift up his back as well. So before opening an infant' s airway, place a rolled towel of your hand closest to his feet beneath his back to support it.
- Then gently tilt his head back. You don' t need to neck.
- Cover both his mouth and node with your mouth. To ventilate, give only small breaths - just enough to make his chest rise.
- If you are having trouble ventilating the infant, his stomach may be distended, limiting chest expansion.
- Don' t relieve gastric distension unless absolutely necessary, because the infant may aspirate stomach contents.
- But if his abdomen is so tense you can' t ventilate, turn him onto his right side and gently press on his epigastric region.
- Gastric distension is caused by delivering too much air, so give only enough air to make the infant' s chest rise.
- Because an infant' s neck is short and chubby, palpate his brachial rather than carotid pulse. The brachial pulse is located on the inside of the upper arm, midway between the shoulder and the elbow.

- Don' t palpate his apical pulse-what you think is a pulse may be just precordial activity.
- To locate your hand position for cardiac compression, draw an imaginary line between the infant's nipples. (An infant' s heart is located higher in the chest than a small child' s or adult' s).
- Place two or three fingers in the middle of this line. Deliver about 100 compressions a minute, giving a breath after every five compression.
- Count to yourself: "One, two, three, four, five" (even though you are alone). Because an infant is so small, one rescuer along can try to resuscitate him.

Unconsciousness

Any interference with the normal functioning of the brain and the nerves brings about loss of consciousness. Level of Consciousness

- Partial (Stupor)
- Complete (coma)

Causes of unconsiousness

- Brain injuries
- Convulsions
- Heat strokes
- Diabetes
- Heart attack
- Epilepsy
- Hemorrhage
- Poisons-eg. Carbon mono-oxide poisoning

Management

- See that there is a supply of fresh air and the air passages are free.
- Take the casualty away form harmful gases
- Watch for symptoms of shock
- Remove false teeth
- Loosen tight clothing up to neck, chest and waist.
- If the breathing has stopped or about to stop, turn

the casualty into the required position and start artificial respiration.

- If breathing is noisy, turn casualty to 3 quarter turn position and support in this position with pillows.
- If breathing is not noisy, let the casualty lie on his back, raise the shoulder slightly with the pillow and turn the head to one side
- Watch continuously for any changes in the condition
- Do not leave the casualty until the medical comes
- Do not give any form of drinks in this condition 1
- On return to consciousness, give little water.

FIRST AID EQUIPMENTS

First aid appliances should be kept in a metal or plastic box, which can be opened and closed easily. The box should be labeled clearly with Red Cross sign and "First Aid" should be written on it.

The box should be kept away from children. As and when the items are consumed, they should immediately be replaced.

Bandages and Slings Applications of Bandages

These are made from flannel, calico, elastic net or special paper, they can be improvised by any of the above material, or from stockings or ties.

Uses of Bandages

- Maintain direct pressure over a dressing to control bleeding.
- Retain dressing and slings in position
- Prevent or reduce swelling.
- Provide support for a limb or joint.
- Restrict movement
- Assist in lifting and carrying casualty.

Guidelines

- Bandages should be applied firm enough to keep dressing and splints in position.

- But not so tight as to cause injury to the part or to impede the circulation of the blood.
- A bluish tinge of the finger or nails may be a danger sign that the bandages are too tight.
- Loss of sensation is an other sign.

Types of Bandages

- Triangular bandages.
- Roller bandages
- Special-such as, many tail or ' T' bandages.

Triangular Bandage

The triangular bandage may be used in nursing for slings to support an arm after injury

Roller Bandages

Roller bandages are used for the following purposes..

- To cover and to retain dressing and splints in position.
- To exercise pressure on a part in order to prevent or to reduce swelling.
- To provide support for a part, sprained or dislocated joint
- To prevent and control haemorrhage
- To restrict movement.
- To correct deformity.

Materials

- Roller bandages are made from strips of different material of varying lengths and widths, according to the part to which they are applied.
- Materials commonly used are flannel, open wove cotton, fast edge cotton, calico, crepe or elastic net.
- Before use, the bandage should be firmly and evenly rolled, either by hand or by machine.
- The parts of the bandage are referred to as the head and the free end to tail.
- Usually, a single roller bandage is used, but for, some certain parts, a double headed roller bandage is required.

- In this, the free ends of two roller bandages are sew together leaving the heads to close together, on the same side of the bandage.
- Most roller bandages are 6 yards long, except the very narrow ones, which are usually, short.
- The width lay according to the part of the body to be bandaged.
- The usual width of the bandages are, 1 Inch to 4 to 6 inches.

Rules for the Application of Roller Bandages

- Use a tightly rolled bandage or the correct width.
- Support the part to be bandaged through out.
- For the forearm, the hand should be prone.
- Always stand in front of the patient except when applying a cape line bandage.
- Bandage a limb in the position in which it is to remain.
- Hold the bandage with the head uppermost and apply the outer surface of the bandage to the part, never unroll more than a few inches of bandage at a time.
- Bandage from within outwards and from below upwards, maintain even pressure throughout.
- Begin the bandage with a firm oblique turn to fix it and allow each successive turn to cover two thirds of the previous one, with the free edges lying parallel.
- Make any reverse or crossing a line on the outer side of the limb, except, when this brings them over a wound or prominence of bone, in which case, they must be on the front of the limb.
- Pad the axilla or groin when bandaging these parts, so that, two of the surfaces of skin do not touch beneath the bandage.
- Finish off with a straight turn above the part, hold in the end and fasten with a safety pin.

Points to be Observed

- The comfort of the patient is the first consideration,

except, when arresting haemorrhage or correcting a deformity.

- Neatness and economy must be considered.
- The bandage should be firm and applied with even pressure throughout.
- The extremities must be carefully watched
- For any signs of swelling or blueness due to interference with circulation by a bandage that is too light.

Terms used in Roller Bandaging

- Simple spiral
- Reverse spiral
- Figure of eight
- Spica Simple spiral Is used for parts which are of uniform thickness, such as, a finger or a wrist. The bandage is applied obliquely round the part, each turn cover two thirds (2/
- Of the proceeding one, and the edges being kept parallel.

It is used for parts which vary in thickness and upon which the bandage of circular turns cannot be tied properly like leg and forearms. One or two simple spiral turns are usually made to carry the bandages to the point at which the spiral can no longer be employed. And then the lower edge of its last spiral is fixed with the thumb about halfway between the mid line and outer surface of the limb.

The bandage is then reversed and brought down and carried round the limb, when another reverse is made immediately above the former one. These reverses are repeated as far as necessary and the bandage completed with one or two. Spiral turns straight round the limb.

Care should be taken and that, each reverse occurs immediately above the previous one, so that, the pattern is even. Each turn should cover two thirds of the preceding one, as in the simple spiral. Is used for bandaging limb and for covering joints. It consists of series of loops, encircling the part in the from of a figure of eight. The upper loops being completely hidden by the successive turns end the lower loops forming the pattern. Each one cover the two thirds of the preceding loop and crossing in the same line.

Is a form of the figure of eight in which one turn is very much large then the other. It is used for joints at right angles to the body. eg: shoulder, groin and thumb.

The Divergent Spica

Is a form of the figure of eight in which the turn go alternately above and below a fixed starting turn ending above, and is used for bend joints, as the elbow or heel.

Bandages for Hand, Wrist, Forearm, Elbow and Arm Hand Bandage

With the pronated, (the palm held downwards) fix the bandage by a turning round the wrist and carry the roll obliquely over the back of the hand to the side of the little finger. Carry the bandage round the palm, encircling the finger with one horizontal turn, so that the lower boarder of the bandage, just touches the root of the nail of the little finger. Carry the bandage one more round the palm and then return obliquely to the wrist. The figure of eight turn round the wrist and hand are repeated until the hand is covered and the bandage is then finished with a spiral turn round the wrist.

Wrist, Forearm, and Upper arm Bandages

The wrist and forearm are bandaged by use of the simple and reverse spiral until the elbow is reached. The figure of eight turn can be so used, as the limb enlarges as an alternative to the reverse spiral turn, if preferred.

Bend the elbow at right angles, lay the outer side of the bandage on the inner side of the joint and take one straight turn carrying the bandage over the elbow tip and round the limb of the elbow. The second turn is made to encircle forearm and the third arm. Each of these turns being made to cover the margins of the first turn. Continue the turns alternately, below and above the first turn, allowing each to cover a little more than two thirds of the previous turn, and finishing about the elbow.

The bandages, as is the forearm, by a succession of reverse spirals or figure of eight turns, and the bandages may be carried on from the forearm, or elbow or started independently, or most conveniently.

Finger Bandages

With the hand pronated, fix the bandage by two circular turns a round the wrist leaving the end free from tying off. Afterwards, carry the bandage obliquely over the back of hand to the base of the finger to be bandaged. Taking the fingers is order, start from the little finger side. Take on spiral turn to the base of the finger nail and then cover the finger by simple spiral turns.

Then carry the bandage a cross the back of the hand to the wrist, and complete it with one straight turn round the wrist. Secure the bandage by a safety pin or by tying the two each of the bandage together. If more than one finger as to be bandaged, take a turn round the wrist between each two fingers and continue as above until the bandage is complete.

Take the bandage straight up to the back of the finger and over the middle of the tip and down the front to the level of the second joint. Holding the turns Back and front with the fingers of the other hand, make two more turns over the tip of the finger, one on either side of the first turn.

Fix the loop with a straight circular turn as near to the tip as possible and then cover the finger by simple spiral turns as before. Being careful to make them from within outwards. Take a straight turn round the wrist and either finish off as before or continue the next finger.

With the hand held, so that, the back of the thumb is upper most, take two turns round the wrist and carry the bandage over the back of the thumb. Encircle the thumb with one or two straight turns, so that, the lower border of the bandage is level with the root of the nail. Carry the bandage back. Over the back of the hand, round the wrist and repeat the figure of eight turns round thumb and wrist, until the wall of the thumb is completely covered. Complete the bandages with one straight turn, round the wrist.

SPICA OF SHOULDER BANDAGE

Place a small pad of cotton wool in each axilla. Take 3- 4 inch bandage and fix it with two spiral turns round the upper part of the arm. Take two or three reverse spiral turns round the upper arm until the bandages reaches the point of the shoulder. Then carry the bandage over the shoulder, across the back and under the opposite armpit.

Bring it back across the chest and arm round under the armpit and over the shoulder again covering two thirds of the previous turn. This form a figure of eight round the arm and the body and the turns are repeated until the whole shoulder is covered. The bandage should be secured by a pin immediately over the injured shoulder.

BANDAGES FOR THE FOOT, ANKLE AND LEG

If the patient is in bed, the heel should be elevated on a support, about 6 inches high. If he is up and about, he should be seated in a chair with the foot supported on a stool or another chair. To avoid stooping, the nurse may, if she prefers, sit opposite to the patient and take his foot on her knee.

Take one or two turns round the ankle to fix the bandage and then take it on obliquely across the foot, the root of the little toe. Make one horizontal turn right round the foot at his level and then carry the bandage back over the foot and take a turn round the ankle just above the heel.

Figure of eight turns are then repeated round the foot and ankle, each turn over lapping the preceding turn by two third of its width, until the whole foot is covered. If the bandage is to be continued up the leg, the reverse spiral or figure of eight turns may be used as for the arm.

The leg should be supported, so that, the heel projects well over the edge of the chair, stool or cushion on which it is placed. The foot should be kept at right angles to the leg. Commence the bandage by a turn over the tip of the heel. The bandage is then carried round the foot just below the tip of the heel, so that, the margin of the bandage covering the tip of the heel is well covered.

It is then brought over the ankle and taken round the leg,

just above the tip of the heel, so that, the other margin of the bandage covering the heel tip is now also covered.

The turns are repeated. Each turn being made just below and above the preceding one until the heel is well covered and the bandage so extends from halfway along the foot to well above the ankle.

Flex the knee, lay the outer side of the bandage against the knee and take one straight turn over the knee cap. The bandage is thus brought round the knee, just below and the just above. Note that the margins of the bandage covering the kneecap are covered as in the elbow and heel bandages. The turns are repeated below and above the joint until the whole knee is covered and the bandage is then secured by one straight turn round the thigh.

Place the outside of the bandage on the inner side of the thigh about 6 inches below the groin. Carry the bandage horizontally round the limb and make three or four ascending reverse spiral turns round the thigh.

Carry the bandages from within outwards over the front of the groin and up round the hip and back, passing over the prominence of the hip bone on the opposite side. Bring the bandage down, over the abdomen to the outer side of the thigh and repeat the figure of eight round the body and the thigh until the hip is covered.

This is applied in the same way as the spica for the hip except that the bandage is started higher up. The reverse spiral and omitted and the crossings are made over the front of the groin instead of on the outer side of the front of the thigh.

Lay the outer surface of the bandage over the right groin from without inwards and pass the bandage round the thigh, carrying it up over the front of the right groin to the left hip. Round the back and right hip and over the lower part of the abdomen to the outer side of the thigh. Pass the bandage under the thigh, up to the left groin round the back and right hip and down again to the inner side of the right hip and down to the inner side of the right thigh. These turns, which really from of double figure of eight, round the body and right thigh and round the body and left thigh, are repeated until both groins as covered each turn being slightly higher than the covering two thirds of the preceding one.

HEAD AND OTHER BANDAGE CAPELINE BANDAGE

The bandage is, sometimes, used when the whole scalp is to be covered. A double headed roller bandage is used. The patient should be seated and the nurse should sand behind the patient. Place a centre of the outer surface of the bandage in the centre of the forehead, the lower border of the bandage lying just above the eyebrows.

The head of the bandage as brought over the temples and above the years to the nape of te neck where the ends are crossed. The upper bandage being carried, round the head and other brought over the centre of the top of the scalp to the root of the nose. The bandage which encircles head is now brought over the forehead, covering and fixing the bandage which could cross the scalp.

This bandage is then brought back over the scalp. Slightly to one side of the centre, thus covering one margin of the original turn. At the back, it is again crossed and fixed by the encircling bandage and is turn back over the scalp to the opposite side of the centerline, now covering the other margin of its original turn.

These backward and forward turns are repeated to alternate side of the centre, each one being, in turn, fixed by the encircling bandage until the whole scalp is covered. The bandages is completed by a circular turn round the head and pinned in the centre of the forehead.

Lay the outer surface of the bandage against forehead and carry the bandage round the head in one circular turn, bandaging away from the injured ear. Towards the sound side, carry the bandage round to the back of the head, low down in the nape of the neck again, repeat these. Each turn being slightly higher than the previous one as it cover the dressing, but slightly over as it cover the hair.

Continue until the whole is covered and complete the bandage by one straight turn around the forehead, pinning where all the turns cross one another some people prefer to take the bandage around the forehead between each turn covering the dressing, but this makes a heavy bulk around the head which is not really necessary.

Lay the outer surface of the bandage against the forehead and take the circular turn round the head, bandaging away from the injured eye. Carry the bandage on, round side for the second time. Take it obliquely to the back of the head, under the prominence at the back of the skull and from there bring it upwards beneath the ear of the affected side, over the pad of the circular turn and continue. Over the head to the starting point. Repeat this turn two or three times until the dressing is covered, finishing with a safety pin just above the good eye.

Many tail bandages are used for abdominal wound certain chest dressing and for any part where the use of a roller bandage would entail a great amount of movement and exertion for the patient. It consists of a number of strips or tails of cotton material, 4-6 inches wide and of sufficient length to encircle the part and overlap at least 8 inches. Each strip overlies the one above by two thirds of its width and the whole is secured in the centre by a piece of the same material. All seams must be sewn so that, there are no hard ridges to hurt the patient.

Bandages for the chest are sometimes provided with two tails, stitched to the top of the back piece and slanting slightly outwards, which pass over the shoulder and are pinned to the front the bandage when the other tails are folded over to keep the bandage from slipping down.

Similarly, abdominal bandages are sometimes provided with two tails stitched to the bottom of back piece and are called groin straps which are passed between the legs and secured to the front of the bandage to prevent it from slipping up. Smaller many tail bandages may sometimes be used to keep a dressing on a limb.

The advantage of the many tail bandage are that, it is easily applied and adjusted and a wound can be inspected without any disturbance to the patient.

The disadvantages are that, if it is applied with little support, it tends to slip and become displaced and can easily be undone by the patient.

The Application of Abdominal Many tail Bandage

For the bandage to be comfortably and efficiently applied, two people are required, although in and emergency one can manage. The patient should be lying quite flat before any attempt is made to apply or adjust a many tail bandage. The bandage is prepared with the tails rolled into the centre, from either end, the smooth portion of the back being uppermost and being placed next to the patient.

The bandage is placed in the position, so that, the centre band lies under the patients back. The bandage is applied from below upwards. One tail being brought across the body at a time and held in position by a tail from the opposite side. The last tail is brought obliquely downwards and secured with a safety pin.

T Bandage

"T" bandages consist of two strips o flannel, about 4 inches wide, stitches together in the form of a "T". The horizontal strip is made long enough to pass round the body and the vertical strip is passed up between the legs. It is then pinned to the horizontal strip to keep rectal of perineal dressing in position.

Plaster bandages may be brought ready- made, such as, the "Gypsona" tape bandage or may be prepared by rubbing dry plaster of paris into the meshes of strip of book muslin. Plaster of paris bandages are used. a. To make splints to immobilize fractures b.

To protect the wound or to immobilize a part to relieve a pain and promote healing. c. To make plaster beds and jackets. The bandages are applied wet and as they dry, they form a hard support to the fracture site. It should be protected from bending or cracking until completely dry and set. A plaster tends to shrink as it dries and if it gets too tight, it may impede circulation.

A patient with a plaster applied to a limb should be

instructed to report back to the hospital immediately if the extremely becomes blue, cold, or swollen.

Adhesive Bandage

In certain circumstances, the doctor may order an adhesive bandage to be worn. These give fine support and may be used for protection and to promote healing in condition, such as, varicose ulcer. Examples of those are elastoplast and crepe bandages. These are supplied according to similar rules to those relating to roller bandages. But great care must be taken to see that the bandage lies smoothly against the skin and that, there are no folds or wrinkles in the bandage.

Tubular Gauze Bandage

This is a special form of tubular bandage, which can be applied with an applicator to any part of the body. It is ideal for small dressing on hands and limbs.

Bandage for the Jaw

Take a narrow strip of material, about 4 feet long or a narrow fold triangular bandage and place the centre of it, under the chin. Carry one end upwards over the top of the head and cross with the other end above the ear. Carry the shorter end low down across the front of the forehead and the larger end in to opposite direction round the back of the head and tie off close, above the other ear.

SLINGS Use of Slings

- To support injured arms.
- To prevent pull by upper limb of injuries to chest, shoulder and the neck.

Types of Slings: The arm Slings

The arm sling is used in cases of fractured ribs, injuries of upper limbs and in cases of fracture in the fore arm, wrist and hands after the application of splints or plaster casts and bandaging.

- Face the casualty, put one end of the spread

triangular bandage over the uninjured shoulder with the point on the injured side.

- Pass the end around the neck and bring it over the injured shoulder. The other end will, now, be hanging down over the chest.
- Place the forearm horizontally across the chest and bring the hanging end up. The forearm is now covered by the bandage.
- Tie the two ends in such a way that the forearm is horizontally or slightly tilted upwards and the knot is placed in the pit, above the collar bone.
- Tuck the part of sling which is loose at the elbow, behind the elbow and bring the fold to the front and pin it up to the front the bandage.
- Place the free base of the bandage in such a way that its margin is just at the base of the nail of the little finger. The nails of all the finger should be exposed.
- Inspect the nails to see, if there is any bluish colour. A bluish colour shows that there is a dangerous tightening of splint or plasters and therefore, free flow of blood is not possible.
- If the casualty is not wearing a coat, place a soft pad under the neck portion of the sling to prevent rubbing of the skin in that place.

Collar and cuff Sling

This sling is used to support the wrist only.

- The elbow is bent and the forearm is placed across the chest in such a way that the fingers touch the opposite shoulder. In this position, the sling is applied
- A clove hitch is passed round the wrist and the ends tied in the hollow above the collar bone on the injured side.
- A triangular sling is used in treating a fracture of the collar bone. It helps to keep the hand raised high up, giving relief from pain due to the fracture.
- Place the forearm across the chest with the fingers

pointing towards the opposite shoulder and the palm over the breast bone.

- Place an open bandage over the chest, with one end over the hand and the point beyond the elbow.
- Tuck the base of the bandage comfortably, under the forearm and hand.
- Fold the lower end, also round the elbow and take it up and cross the back over the uninjured shoulder and tie it with the other free hand into the hollow, above the collar bone.
- Tuck the point between forearm and bandage.
- Tuck the fold, so formed, backwards over the lower half of the arm and fix it with a safety pin.

First aid in Disasters

Disasters are sudden, catastrophic events that disturb patterns of life in which there is possible loss of life and property in addition to multiple injuries. The disasters means an adverse or unfortunate event or great and sudden misfortune. The common elements of any disaster are casualties, homeless person disturbance of sanitary facility, some degree of panic and need for emergency medical services.

Types of Disaster

- Natural disaster - Flood or drought, windstorm, (cyclone or hurricane) earthquake or volcanic eruption, epidemic
- Man-made unintentional disasters: Fire, explosions, and accidents of trains, aircraft or ships
- Intentional disasters: Ordinary bombing, atomic bombing, biological warfare and chemical warfare

Responsibilities of Nurses in disaster

- During disaster the sick person need ingenuity, and the nurse should have imagination to utilize things that are available at hand.
- She should give constant observation and treatment to seriously wounded person to arrest the bleeding and should save the life.

- She should check the infection. 4. She should maintain the sanitation and cleanliness
- She should arrange the initial examination and health checkup. 6. Arrange for food facilities to the injured.
- Arrange them for clean drinking water.
- Arrange for transportation.
- She should make arrangement to intimate the relative as early as possible.

Community Emergencies

- Fire explosion: It is the commonest disaster seen in the community.
- Flood: This disaster is commonly seen during the rainy season and the people loving near seas side or low lying areas
- Earthquakes: It occurs without prior significance
- Famine: Famine is the disaster caused by the nature.

Handling and Transport Leading a Stretcher

Five people will be required to load a casulity into a stretcher, four to life the causality and one to move the stretcher position of the helpers for manual lift.

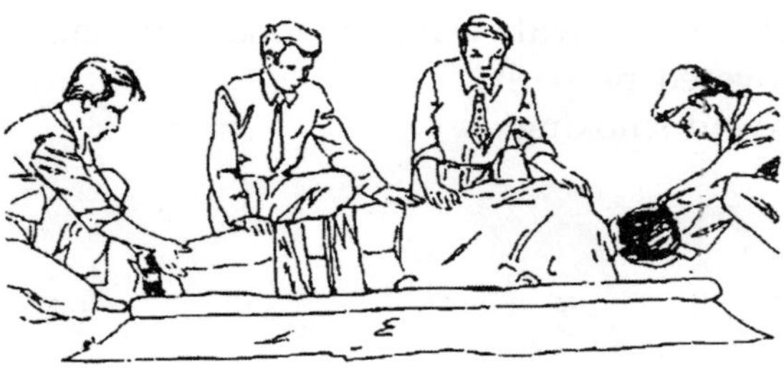

Fig. Leading to a stretcher Manual lift. If the causality has a fractured spine. Do not move him unless absolutely necessary.

Carrying a stretcher. Unless casulaity is suffering from shock the head should be kept higher than the chest. As a general rule the casualty should be carried feet first. Loading Ambulance: The trolly bed should be loaded and unloaded carefully.

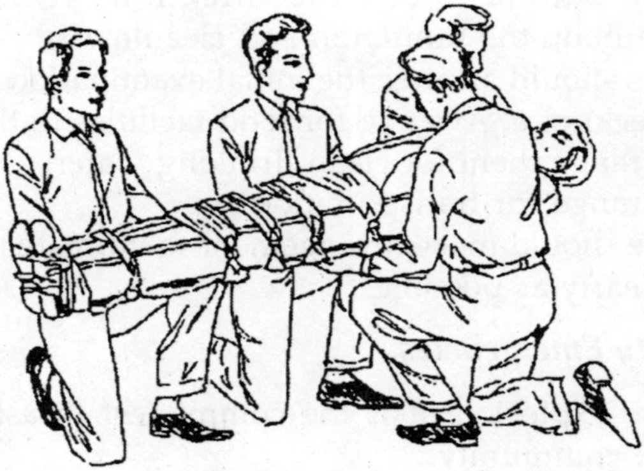

Fig. Manual lift for a fractured spine.

Promoting safety Consciousness in Community Safety at home

The house should be built as strong and durable. The safety measures have to be followed.

- Avoid stain of oil, grease etc.
- Bathroom should not be slippery.
- Electrical appliances should not be touched with wet hands.
- Children should not have access to match box.
- The vessel with water or food materials should be covered properly.
- Avoid smoking

Chapter 10

Health Management

DEFINITION OF HEALTH

The World Health Organisation defines health as "a state of complete, physical, mental, and social wellbeing, and not merely the absence of disease or infirmity". It may also be defined as "able to live most and serve best". Health in general is a value asset, though often one does not realise the value until it is lost through illness. Health influences one's way of life. It improves personal efficiency and helps the individual in the attainment of most of his personal goals.

EFFECTIVE HEALTH MANAGEMENT

In order to attain the highest level of effective health system, awareness on the importance of the health education and sustained practices of the said guidelines is the most important component in the health care delivery system for all.

Definition of Health Education

The World Health Organisation defines health education as the "sum total of all the experiences, which favourably influence knowledge, skills, attitudes and practices of all individuals towards his personal and community health". Health Education may also be defined as a process of change within the human organism, which is related to personal, and community health goals.

According to Alma-Ata declaration "Health education is a process aimed at encouraging people to want to be healthy to know how to stay healthy to do what they can individually and collectively to maintain health and seek help when needed". Health education is the act of getting people to do something for themselves to attain better health.

The nurse should remember that the practice of health education is not merely a simple speech needed only for ignorant people, but it is applied for all, rich and poor, young and old, educated and illiterate, sick and health individuals at all times, especially when they have "felt needs" for health. Health education involves teaching about reducing health risk factors, increasing a person' s level of wellness and taking specific protective health measures.

Aims and Objectives of Health Education

- To help people to develop an awareness of health needs and problems.
- To acquire knowledge and skills on matters related to health and health resources.
- To develop desirable attitudes towards personal and community health and to solve their health problems by their own actions and efforts.
- To participate and co-operate with health workers and use health services for their maximum benefit.
- To adopt the altered health and function.

Principles of Health Education

Some basic principles that should be followed while giving health education.

- Interest - The interest of the individual or the group should be considered. For example a patient may want to know more about his illness rather than facts about environmental hygiene.
- Acceptable - It should be acceptable to the people as well as the leaders of the community. People's customs, beliefs, traditional habits and ways of living must be considered. For example vegetarians should not be advised to take meat. beliefs, traditional habits and ways of living must be considered. For example vegetarians should not be advised to take meat.

- *Practicable*: It should be practicable. Consider the educational level, income of the family, capacity to understand and the mental make up. For example, asking the mother with a poor income to take plenty of milk or meat is meaningless.
  Similarly asking her to take lettuce a leafy vegetable that is not commonly available or used in this country will not be practicable. Also asking the mother to take plenty of iron, calcium and protein will not mean much to her, instead of which, mentioning foods rich in the above nutrients will be more helpful.
- *Participation*: This is usually done by allowing free discussion.
- *Known to unknown*: One should start teaching the learners from what they already knew and then explain the new knowledge.
- *Reinforcement*: Repetition helps learning, Facts and points should be repeated frequently as it assists better memory and understanding.
- *Motivation*: Motivation is another important factor to bear in mind while teaching. The desire to learn, change or modify the behaviour of the learner must be created.
- *Demonstration*: This is showing people exactly what to do by practical ways.
- Learning by doing - Allow the individual to learn to do things by himself. Give sufficient time to practice when possible.
- *Establish good inter-personal relationship*: This should start from the very beginning. The nurse should not be over - anxious or disrespectful even when eating with illiterate and poor people. Allow the groups or individuals to express their view and clear their doubts.
- Adequate planning is essential even if it is a five-minute talk.
- Health education should be carried out with the cooperation of the other staff in the department and

in the community with the help of the local leaders, school teachers, dais etc.

Content and Scope of Health Education

Content of health education varies according to the situation and is vast in practice. The content of health education may be classified as follows:

- *Human*: Normal structure and function of the body etc.
- *Nutrition*: Nutrition needs at all ages, health and illness prevention of deficiency disease etc. Selection and cooking of food for health.
- *Hygiene*: Personal and environmental hygiene and ways of healthfull living. Regular health examinations, early correction of defects, protection of water and safe disposal of refuse.
- *Family Welfare Service*: Family health, family planning, child care, maternal care etc.
- *Control of Communicable Disease*: Disease causing organisms, mode of entry, prevention of spread, treatment and control of communicable disease, role of immunization etc.
- *Mental Health*: Maintenance of mental health, Healthy attitudes
- *School health*: Personal hygiene, good food, prevention of communicable diseases etc.
- Prevention of accidents in homes - Hospitals, school and industries, Health hazards due to physical, biological and mechanical causes and ways to prevent them.
- *Use of health service:* Where available, when and how to make use of services.

APPROACHES OF HEALTH EDUCATION

Regulatory Approach

There are occasions when people are indifferent to their own health thus endangering the health of the community, in which case the regulatory or legal approach seeks to protect the health of the public through the enforcement of laws and regulations. The nurse and other health workers must be aware of all these laws, eg. Primary vaccination against small-pox is compulsory in India.

Servicing Approach

This is mainly the responsibility of the health department and health workers both in government and non-government health agencies.

The service or administrative approach aims at providing all the health facilities needed by the community so that the people will make use of them in order to improve their own health. The service approach will be a failure when it is not based on the "felt needs" of the people. Hence all health workers must find out the problems and needs of the people before teaching and providing care to them.

Educational Approach

The educational approach is considered as one of the important means for bringing about changes in the health practices of people and helping them to recognise their health need. It involves proper communication and motivation of the community to make the right decision in order to attain health. Though it is a good method, it is a slow perseverance to have permanent and enduring results. However small it may be, educational approach may be classified as follows:

Individual Approach

This is usually done by the health worker (nurse) wherever and whenever she comes in contact with individuals who need knowledge, guidance and counselling regarding individual health problems and needs. Personal interviews can be planned or unplanned. Individual health teaching can be done in the hospitals, homes and any health care institutions. In order to teach individuals, we must develop skills and have sufficient knowledge to gain the confidence of the people (learners).

First of all the nurse should set a good example by practicing principles of healthy living. Example is a good method of teaching. She should practise good health habits such as regular exercises, rest, sleep, personal cleanliness, wearing clean uniforms, washing hands after touching infected materials and before eating and so on.

Good food, safe water and good food habits are essential to promote, maintain and prevent deficiency diseases. It is important that she gives major consideration to the selection, cooking and eating of proper foods. Safe and clean environment is necessary wherever we live and work.

Cleanliness is next to godliness and all health workers should maintain cleanliness and have proper disposal of waste and refuse. This will help in the prevention and spreading of diseases to a great extent. Often in busy hospitals, health centers, clinics etc., one may not find much time of frequency planned health teaching programmes. Therefore the nurse must bear in mind that incidental teaching is an on-going process and she should be on the lookout for health teaching opportunities.

For example while giving patient care she should make health education an essential component. It may be about personal hygiene, balanced food or how to prevent certain diseases etc.

Teaching may be given to patient's relatives and friends. Teaching may be given to patient's illness and how they can help the patient during and after the period of illness. Health teaching is also useful to individual hospital workers (Class IV staff).

They should be helped in maintaining a clean and safe environment in order to prevent hospital cross infection and spread of communicable disease. The nurse should teach and supervise the workers in the collection and disposal of waste, collection of soiled linen, washing of hands of those attending to the toilet of patients, washing bed pans etc.

Family Approach

The family is an important unit of society, and individual

problem affects the whole family. They are often emotionally involved and much worried about the individual who is suffering. Usually much can be done during home visit. Family members can be taught how to look after the sick, how to prevent home accidents, food budgeting and planning, care of the children, care of the pregnant mothers, family welfare services (family planning), immunization and all about personal and environmental sanitation.

Group Approach

This is usually organized to teach small groups, which will facilitate discussion, exchange of ideas and clearing of doubts after the teaching is over for a short period. Better results are achieved when groups of people with similar interest are selected for example, patients with similar problems, interest and needs.

Also needs of school children, adolescents, industrial worker, mothers and fathers will be different, and they may be taken separately. The health worker should plan well ahead of time or organization groups in the wards, clinics and community centers at a convenient place and time suitable to them. Suitable audio visual aids must be selected to have good results.

TEACHING OF PATIENTS

The choice of what to teach the patient is based on:

- What we know about the patient; information gained by study of the chart, doctor's comments, conversation with the patient.
- The patient's physical conditions: even seriously ill patients learn from your attitude. Example Cleanliness, need for emergency, etc.
- The interest of the patient: at first most likely to be interested in his disease - what he needs to know to get well, to live with residual condition to prevent relapse and to help others to avoid it.
- Secondary interests: knowledge of use to his family or general interest.

- Patient' s intelligence: some are able to learn on a higher level than others.
- Probable ability to apply teaching.
- Facts for immediate use - not something vague for future.
- Material related to local customs.
- Nurse's knowledge: thorough preparation. 10) Consultation with notes, texts and senior staff, so that the nurse thoroughly understands the material herself. She should not try to teach in advance of her own knowledge.

HOW TO TEACH THE PATIENT

By Quoting Example

The nurse's personal appearance, the conscience with which she carries out her work, his/her attention to sanitation and health rules and other good health practices will be observed and followed by the patients.

By Telling

The nurse must establish a good relationship for teaching between patient and him/her and must gain the patient's confidence. She/he should use simple language, avoiding foreign or technical words, and teach only one or two facts at a time, choosing the most important. Stress should be laid on positive action, especially on the DO' s rather than on the DON'T' s.

By showing: "One look is Worth a Thousand Words"

Demonstrate to the patient by actually doing. Show the article you are talking about, the kind he would use at home. Let him touch it or hold it. Explain what you are doing and why. When possible let the patient demonstrate in return. Use pictures, flash-cards, books, sample articles or models,

By Reviewing: "Repetition teaches"

Ask the patient to tell you what you have taught, both at

the end of the conversation and the next day. Make any corrections or additions if necessary. Allow the patient to tell facts that are right.

By Approving

Give praise and recognition for learning of making improvements.

TEACHING SMALL GROUPS

- *Plan materials*: Gather illustrative material know subject thoroughly and have objective in teaching, Consult senior nurses, staff and text books.
- *Plan groups*: Select time in advance, notify all concerned. Select people with common interest. Keep Group small. Sit in circle.
- *Method*: Gain interest with pictures, models or leading questions. Teach subject in simple language for about 5 minutes. Use visual aids, black board, pictures, sample etc. Look at each person while talking. Permit and encourage questions and comments. Keep to the subject but do not stifle other questions - refer to them another time. Let one of the groups participates as a module, but avoid possible embarrassment. Practical demonstrations may be given by each group.

Role playing: acting out an imaginary scene, may be used occasionally. Try to leave behind something definite to do with the group. Review and sum up the teaching at the end of the class.

- *Teaching Mass*: refers to educating large groups of people by using the mass media. There is no two-way communication and the results are not very encouraging but useful, especially when health information has to be given to the community, e.g. drinking of boiled water during floods, family planning services etc.

METHODS COMMONLY USED

- *Group Discussion*: (a) Symposium b) Panel discussion.

It is a two-way communication. People learn by exchanging their view and experience. Small groups of 8 to 12 are more effective and active, Participation of member is encouraged.

- *Lecture method*: It is one-way method of teaching but it can be made more meaningful by use of audio-visual aids and discussions.
- Questions and Answers method (Socratic method): This method is suitable both for individuals and groups. Learning takes place through questions and answers.
- *Demonstration method*: The purpose of demonstration is to show how to do something. Demonstration must be done using simple equipment available and familiar to the learner (patient).
- *Role play*: This is based on the assumption that many values in a given situation cannot be expressed in words, and the communication can be made more effective if the situation is dramatized by the group.
- *Project method*:
  - It requires activity and gives a sense of accomplishment. Subjects are organised into units that can be dealt with by a student or learner group.
  - Project assignment is adaptable to community health in which the learner works together in groups.
- Workshop and conference - adopted to professional groups, teachers etc. The group works together to explore all aspects of a subject and to reach specific goals.

AUDIOVISUAL AIDS

Audiovisual aids play an important role in health education, They can be classified into three groups - purely auditory aids, purely visual and a combination of both auditory and visual aids. Media or materials in health education can be used for different purposes and for different groups of people. Learning and understanding seems to result when more senses, such as, touch, sight, and hearing are reached by the media. If used properly they create interest and motivate people to learn. Learning is made more permanent because these aids supply a concrete basis for learning rather than abstract thinking.

TYPES OF AIDS

For Mass Media

- Motion picture
- Film strips
- Exhibition
- Radio
- Television
- Mass media

Other Aids

- Black board
- Bulletin board
- Flannel graph or Khadigraph

The cut out pictures in bright colours should be pasted on to sand paper or on to some rough material and the same are fixed on to flannel boards while teaching.

Practice before you teach for, if done well, it holds the attention of the learners. The theme of story should be selected in advance and the figures kept in order to be used without delay.

- *Flash cards*: They are pictures arranged in sequence, which illustrate a story. Support the cards on your chest wall and practice in order to make your teaching effective. Use a pointer so that the picture is not covered by your hand.
- *Posters*: Posters should be colourful to catch the eye and convey the message clearly. Simple language and short sentences should be used. If used in the clinic, outpatients department or health centers, they should be changed frequently. When possible explain the

message to the learners and use them to supplement your health teaching.

- *Suspense charts*: Each section of the chart is covered and is exposed one by one to reveal the story or ideas without exposing the whole chart at a time.
- *Puppets*: Puppets are dolls made by hand and a story can be narrated using them. It is a popular teaching aid to health teaching, both children and adults enjoy seeing pupper shows.

SELECTION AND USES OF AUDIOVISUAL AIDS

Uses of Printed Teaching Material

The following criteria are guides for the selection of the books and other printed teaching materials. How each applies in a given instance depends upon the specific teaching objectives, which have been set up to meet particular needs.

Criteria for Selecting audio Visual aids.

- The facts should be scientifically accurate.
- Needed materials should be present
- All the information should be pertinent.
- It should cover the entire requirements.
- All the ideas should be essential, significant and important to clear understanding.

Chapter 11

Principles and Practices of Nursing

Much ill-health and the majority deaths in India are due to:

- Lack of cleanliness, leading to spread of infection.
- Poor nutrition, leading to poor resistance to disease.

Personal cleanliness and public cleanliness are necessary for health of the community. At the same time good nutrition helps to prevent sickness and helps the sick persons to fight against the diseases. But many people in India do not have money to buy good food. They struggle to obtain food for themselves and their families.

More over, there are many other living organisms big and small, competing with each other and live with people for food. These living organisms include germs and parasites, which attack our bodies. Some take nutrients from us and others live on our blood. These microorganisms cause serious disease that leads to death.

INFECTIONS

When the living microorganisms enter and attack our bodies causing sickness, it is called infection. Most organisms can live only inside man or animal, and they go from one to another, spreading disease. Many are so small that they may be seen only by means of microscope.

Micro-Organisms

Classifications of Microorganisms

- Pathogenic organisms:Pathogenic organisms are those, which produce disease.

- Nonpathogenic organisms: Non-pathogenic organisms are those, which break down the refusal and sewage, and those, which help in making curds, cheese, bread and alcohol. There are four main groups of microorganisms.
- Bacteria include cocci, bacilli, spirella and spirochaetes
- Fungi are plant like organisms and include yeast. Yeast are useful for making bread and wine. Penicillin also is produced from the yeast. Some fungi are pathogenic and cause diseases such as ringworm and oral thrush.
- Protozoa are animal type of organisms,. They are much bigger than bacteria. Examples: malaria parasite causes the malaria fever and the entamoeba hystelytica causes dysentery.
- Viruses are smaller than bacteria. It can pass through the finest filters. They cannot be seen through an ordinary microscope, but only through an electron microscope. Common viral infections are common cold, measles, chickenpox, smallpox, rabies and poliomyelitis.

Entry of Infection into Human Body

- Organisms may enter the body in one of the three ways
- Digestive tract- swallowed in food or water.
- Respiratory tract - breathed in with air.
- Skin and mucus membranes - through a wound, weakened surface or injection.

Organisms leave the body of an infected person in the following ways.

- Excreta - faeces and urine.
- Coughing, sneezing and sputum.
- Pus and wound discharges.
- Blood, eg mosquito bites and injection needle.

Each type of organisms has its own special path for leaving an infected person and going into a healthy person. Examples are as follows.

Faecal to Oral Route

Faeces may contain:

- Intestinal parasites or ova of worms.
- Amoeba causing dysentery.
- Bacteria causing cholera, typhoid fever or dysentery.
- Viruses of polio or hepatitis.

From the faeces, the organisms may get into drinking water. Flies and dirty hands act as carriers and spread infection by oral route. Children may suck the dirty fingers and organisms enter the body.

Faecal to oral route infection can be prevented by means of:

- Hand washing before preparing or eating food.
- Eating only clean food, kept free from flies.
- Getting rid of flies and breeding places.
- Protecting the water supply and drinking boiled water.
- Use of latrines, or covering the faeces with earth.
- Proper hand washing with soap after defecation.

Faeces to Skin

Hookworm ova passed in faeces, hatch into larvae on the ground. Then the larvae can bite through the skin, usually through bare feet and grow into adult worms in the intestines. Hookworm disease can be prevented if people use latrines and wear slippers.

The tetanus bacillus lives in the intestines of man and animals and is present in cowdung and soil. It enters into the body through a wound or a new born baby' s umbilical cord. The best way to prevent tetanus is by immunization with tetanus toxoid.

Droplet Infection (air Borne)

When a person with infection such as a common cold or tuberculosis, coughs, sneezes or even talks, with his breat organisms are thrown into the air in very small drops of sputum. The droplets may dry up, leaving an infectious dust on clothes, floors and furniture. When another person breathes in or inhales the infection affects the later. The diseases, which are spread by droplet infections, are diphtheria, mumps, measles, chickenpox, smallpox, whooping cough, pneumonia and upper respiratory tract infections. Droplet infection is difficult to prevent. Prevention of droplet infections are:

- Breathe fresh air and avoid crowded places.
- Have sufficient nutritious food.
- Cover the nose and mouth when coughing.
- Persons with tuberculosis should take proper treatment.
- Those with measles, chicken pox, diphtheria etc should be isolated.
- Immunizations especially to protect children.

Upper Respiratory Infections

The upper respiratory system is the part above the trachea, Common respiratory infections (U.R.I) include, the common cold, influenza, or FLU, pharyngitis and tonsillitis. They tend to spread rapidly within 1 to 6 days of incubation period Viruses cause common cold and FLU. Getting cold or wet do not cause these sickness but they may be made worse by getting wet.

Signs and Symptoms

- Dry, sore throat
- Sneezing
- Running or blocked nose.
- Headache, fever and cough.
- Pains in the joints (in the flu)

The symptoms may last for few days. In babies and young children if not treated properly they may lead to complications such as pneumonia, bronchitis etc.

Treatment and Nursing Care

- Bed rest and warmth.
- Plenty of liquids to drink. Orange juice or lemonade are helpful.
- Aspirin tablets may be given. Antibiotics do not help in virus infections.

- Steam inhalation helps to clear a blocked nose. Decongestant nasal drops may be prescribed.
- The nose should be cleaned frequently. Warn people not to sniff or blow the nose vigorously.

Tonsillitis

This may be a symptom of cold or flu, or it may be a bacterial infection of the tonsils.

Signs and Symptoms

- Red swollen tonsils
- Draining pus from the tonsils.
- Fever,
- Pain in the throat
- Difficulty in swallowing.
- Cough with some sputum and vomiting.
- Enlarged lymph glands under the jaw

Treatment and Nursing Care

- Aspirin tablets may be prescribed to relieve the pain.
- Tablets penicillin or penicillin injections if there is bacterial infection.
- Warm saline gargles (one teaspoon salt added to a tumbler of warm water)
- If there is no improvement in 3 days, or if a gray membrane is seen on the tonsils (sign of diphtheria), the patient must

be referred to a doctor.

Pneumonia

This is an acute infection of the lungs caused by bacteria or viruses. When the infection affects both the bronchi and lungs, it is known as bronchopneumonia. Pneumonia is often a complication of measles, whooping cough, asthma or upper respiratory tract infection (U.R.I) and is especially dangerous in children.

Signs and Symptoms

- Rapid, shallow breathing, sometimes with wheezing.

- Nasal flaring
- Cough with sputum, which might be blood stained or with yellowish mucus.
- Fever.
- There may be cyanosis.

Treatment and Nursing Care

- Tablet Penicillin or injection Ampicillin for 5 days.
- Plenty of liquids including water.
- Aspirin will help to reduce fever.
- Support the head and shoulders with pillows, and turn position every hour.
- Steam inhalations may be given to relieve cough and loosen bronchial secretions.

Preventive and Control Measures

- Never neglect a common cold.
- Avoid over crowding
- Sleep in a well ventilated room
- Educate mothers to burp babies after giving feeds
- When a child has measles, whooping cough etc, try to prevent pneumonia by proper treatment and care.
- If pneumonia develops start treatment as quickly a possible.
- The sputum of the patients should be carefully discarded after proper disinfection.

Mumps

This is a virus infection of the parotid glands (parotitis). The source of infection is the saliva and it is spread by droplet infection or fomite.

Signs and Symptoms

- Symptoms usually begin 2 or 3 weeks after contact with an infected person
- Mild fever
- Pain on opening the mouth or eating.
- Difficulty in swallowing (dysphagia)

- A soft swelling appears below the ears at the angle of the jaw. It may affect unilaterally or bilaterally.
- The swelling usually resolves in about 10 days with out any treatment.

Treatment and Nursing Care

- Bed rest
- Tablet Aspirin can be given for pain and fever.
- Give plenty of water etc to drink
- Soft food for easy digestion
- Ice packs or cold wet clothes may be applied to help reduce pain and swelling.
- If signs of meningitis appear (high fever, confusion, irritation convulsion) get medical help immediately.

Prevention and Control

Isolate the infected person from others

Complications:

- Sterility
- Meningitis

Tuberculosis (TB)

This is a chronic infectious disease caused by the tubercle bacillus. When the infected person coughs, droplets of his sputum go into the air and are breathed in by healthy persons. If a person has immunity against the disease, he may get only a primary lesion in the lung, which may heal without treatment. In others, especially children and those who are weak and poorly nourished and people with low immunity, the disease affects and manifest the signs and symptoms of tuberculosis.

Tuberculosis usually affect the lungs (pulmonary tuberculosis). Sometimes it may attack other parts of the body such as the lymph glands in the neck, intestines, uterus, bones brain etc.

Signs and Symptoms of Pulmonary Tuberculosis

- Loss of weight.

- Cough with sputum
- Mild fever in the evening, and sweating at night.
- Fatigue
- Chest pain
- Dyspnoea (difficulty in breathing)
- Haemoptysis (spitting of blood in sputum

Diagnosis

- Sputum smear for acidfast bacilli (AFB)
- X ray chest.

Treatment and Nursing Care

The drugs used in the treatment of Tuberculosis are:

- Injection Streptomycin
- Tablet Isoniazid (1. N. H)
- Tablet Rifamycin
- Tablet Thiacetazone.

T.B germs do not die easily. They will be killed only with continued specific treatment for a prescribed time. Besides the anti tuberculosis treatment (ATT) as above, it is also important to:

- Advice to eat a balanced diet rich in proteins and vitamins as well as energy foods.
- Advice to have enough rest and sleep. It is best to avoid heavy work and doing things that cause fatigue.

Preventive and Control Measures

- Early diagnosis and immediate treatment to prevent the spread of infection.
- Screen the whole family for identifying infection.
- Vaccinate the children with B.C.G.
- The infected person should be isolated from others
- The infected person should cover his mouth when coughing and use a covered cup to receive the sputum.
- He should burn the sputum or dispose it in a safe way.

- Educate the community as to how the infection can be prevented
- Inform that the facilities are available for diagnosis and treatment at free of cost in government hospitals.

Waterborne and Food Borne Disease

Typhoid Fever.

This is a serious disease caused by the typhoid bacillus. The bacteria are swallowed with contaminated food and water. The bacteria.

Flourish in the Payers patches (Lymphoid tissue) of small intestine where ulceration develops. The incubation period is 1 to 3 weeks.

Signs and Symptoms

- High fever, which continues for more than a week.
- Coated tongue
- Headache and malaise
- A comparatively slow pulse (bradycardia) (Pulse rate is usually faster with other types of fever)
- Constipation or diarrhea.
- The abdomen may become swollen and tender,
- Rashes in the abdomen

Diagnosis:

- Widal test
- Blood culture
- Presence of typhoid bacilli in the stools.

Treatment and Nursing Care

- Bed rest
- Capsule Chloromphenical will be given as per prescription.
- Soft nutritious food (non-residual diet)
- Plenty of fluids.
- Careful observation of vital signs,
- Watch for complications such as internal hemorrhage or intestinal perforation.

- Before discharge, the stool test must be negative; otherwise the patient will be a carrier of the disease.

Preventive and Control Measures

- Early identification and proper treatment
- Isolate the patient,
- Disinfect stools, urine and soiled articles.
- Immunise the contact persons with typhoid vaccine.
- Make sure about safe drinking water, safe food especially milk and milk products and control of flies

CHOLERA

This is an acute communicable disease, caused by Vibrio Cholera.

The incubation period is from a few hours to 2 days. The organisms are swallowed with contaminated food and water. In the small intestine they quickly multiply and produce a toxin which causes the intestinal wall to secrete a great deal of water and salts.

Signs and Symptoms

- Severe diarrhea and vomiting (the stools looks like rice water)
- Severe dehydration
- The pulse is very weak and rapid and blood pressure is low (hypotension).
- The infected person complains of severe thirst
- Painful cramps in legs and abdomen.
- Sunken eyes
- Urine output is low (oliguria),
- In severe conditions the infected patient may collapse

Diagnosis

A patient with rice-water stools should be suspected of having cholera. A stool specimen should be collected and sent immediately to the laboratory for confirmation of diagnosis.

Treatment and Nursing Care

- Isolate the infected person from others immediately

- Rehydrate the patient with adequate intravenous fluids
- Administer antibiotics as per doctors prescription
- Monitor vital signs (pulse respiration, temperature and blood pressure) every hour
- Watch for the urine output
- The patient should be encouraged to take rice congee, buttermilk and plenty of oral fluids to replace fluid loss.
- If a child is breast fed, feeds should be continued

Preventive and Control Measures

- Surveillance- investigation of all cases of diarrhoea.
- Immediate notification of suspected cases.
- Isolation of the patient, with special care to disinfect stools, and vomit
- If a person dies, the body should be wrapped in a sheet soaked in 2per cent Lysol and disposed off by burning.
- Sanitation measures
  - Chlorination of all water sources,
  - Advice to drink boiled water and
  - Safe food practice (food hygiene) - protected from flies and proper hand washing.
- Immunise the community with cholera vaccine during an outbreak of cholera.
- Educate the community on ways of preventing cholera.

Infectious Hepatitis

This is a viral that affects the liver. It often comes on epidemic. The virus enters the body through contaminated water and food. The incubation period is 15 to 20 days.

Signs and Symptoms

- Loss of appetite,
- Nausea and vomiting

  Fever and fatigue

- Mild abdominal pain
- Hepatomegaly (enlarged liver)
- Yellowish discoloration of conjunctiva
- Urine turns to dark yellow

Treatment and Nursing Care

- Complete bed rest
- Advise to drink a lot of liquids rich in glucose, vitamins and minerals (Orange, sugarcane, lemon juice, glucose water etc)
- Antibiotics and other drugs are not advised in treatment of infectious hepatitis as they may cause more damage to the liver.
- Easily digestible - fat and protein free diet should be given

Preventive and Control Measures

- The sick person' s stools must be carefully disposed of to avoid spread of disease.
- The person attending the patient must wash hands well after each contact to prevent cross infection.
- Safe drinking water and better sanitation will help to get rid of infectious hepatitis from the community.

ACUTE GASTROENTERITIS

It is an acute diarrheal disease caused by bacterial infection, or sometimes due to a viral infection. The incubation period is 1-7 days. It may be as short as 6 hours.

Signs and Symptoms

- Sudden onset of diarrhoea (watery stools)
- Abdominal cramps.
- Nausea and vomiting
- Mild fever.
- Dehydration may be severe.

Treatment and Nursing Care

- If there is a delay in getting medical aid, the nurse should try to prepare oral rehydration fluid as follows.

- Boiled water, 1 liter (4 cups)
- Glucose powder 20gms or 8 level teaspoons.
- Common salt (Sodium chloride) 2 gm or ½ level teaspoon.
- Baking soda (Sodium bi-carbonate) 2 gm or ½ level teaspoon.
- Potassium chloride, 1½ gm or ½ level teaspoons.

- The amount of fluid loss must be replaced, either by mouth or by intravenous fluids immediately.

Adults and older children should have plenty of clear fluids such as coconut water, sweetened tea without milk etc. As the patient recovers, a bland diet with well-boiled rice, biscuits, etc may be given.

- Babies may have rice water or oral rehydration fluid in small sips and every 5 to 10 minutes and should continue feeding.
- Antibiotics such as ampicillin or tetracycline may be given as per doctor' s prescription.

Preventive and Control Measures

- Isolation and strict rules to prevent cross- infection in hospitals.
- Maintain cleanliness of food, water and milk.
- Fly control, and protection of food.
- Breastfeeding for babies. If the baby is fed with formula feeds, fluids and all utensils used must be boiled.
- Sanitary disposal of faces.

Dysentery

It is an infectious disease in which the patient passes stools with mucus and blood. The infectious microorganisms enter the body through the contaminated food and water and causes inflammation of the bowels. It may be bacillary dysentery or amoebic dysentery.

A. Bacillary Dysentery

It is caused by bacteria which are swallowed in food,

water or milk contaminated through flies or by direct contact with faeces of infected persons. It may occur in epidemics. It is dangerous in infants and in very old people.

The incubation period is 1-7 days.

Signs and Symptoms

- Fever, vomiting and abdominal pains.
  The patient always wants to have a motion
- Blood stained and mucous stool is passed.
- There may be dehydration.
- There is an urge to pass stools always

Diagnosis

- A stool specimen for microscopic study to identify the causative organisms.

Treatment and Nursing Care

- Replace fluid loss by oral rehydration fluid.
- Infants should continue breast feeding.
- The doctor may order Antibiotics.

Preventive and Control Measures

- Isolation of patient, and disinfections of faces and soiled articles.
- Sanitary disposal of faeces.
- Safe drinking water.
- Fly control and protection of food.
- Food hygienic especially in preparing and handling food

AMOEBIC DYSENTERY

It is caused by a parasite called Entamoeba Hystalytica. It enters the body through contaminated food and water.

The incubation period is 3 to 4 weeks.

Signs and Symptoms

- Blood and mucus passed in large stools alternating with constipation.

- Dull pain on the right side of the abdomen.
- The persons will become anaemic
- Sometimes there is an acute attack of diarrhea.
- The infected person may develop liver abscess.

Diagnosis

It is by the presence of E.H amoebae or cysts in a fresh (warm) specimen of faces examined with a microscope.

Treatment and Nursing Cure

- Tablet Metroniadazole as per prescription.

Preventive and control measures

- Same as given for bacillary dysentery,
- Carriers should be identified and treated

Poliomyelitis

This is also called infantile paralysis because it more often affects children and causes paralysis. It is caused by a virus, which enters the body through contaminated food and water and attacks the nerves. The incubation period 4-7 days,

Most children are infected with poliovirus at sometime, but most of them have no symptoms. Some children have a few days of fever and painful muscles and then recover. Some get a meningeal type of which lasts a few days and they recover in most cases.

Signs and Symptoms

- Polio is usually recognized only when the child stops walking and one of the legs are weak.
- Before this manifestation the child may have had a cold and fever, neck stiffness and mild diarrhoea for a few days.
- Paralysis may affect one or both legs, arms and in severe cases also the diaphragm causing difficulty with breathing.
- The paralysis stops getting worse when the fever stops.

- Some patients' recover completely in about 6 weeks, but many are left with permanent paralysis and perhaps deformity.

Treatment and Nursing Care

- There is no specific treatment for poliomyelitis.
- If the child has pain, give him aspirin, or paracetemol.

NO Injections are Allowed

- The infected person should be kept at bed rest with the affected limb supported, and splinted if necessary.
- After 10 days the mother should be taught to do passive exercise for five minutes for 5 times a day.
- If paralysis continues, arrange for physiotherapy.

Preventive and Control Measures

- Oral polio vaccine (O.P.V) for all infants and children according to the National Immunisation Schedule:
- Sanitary latrines and safe drinking water for all.
- Isolation of cases and disinfection.
- Search for polio cases especially among children.
- During an epidemic, avoid surgery of children' s nose and throat, and avoid D.P.T vaccine (Diptheria polio and tetanus) immunization.

Medical and Surgical Asepsis

Asepsis means absence of disease producing organisms. The microorganisms of different types are present everywhere in our environment and in the human body. The purpose of medical asepsis is to prevent by all means of cross-infections from one patient to another, including communicable disease infections. The purpose of surgical asepsis is to prevent by all means of infections of the wounds of surgical patients, infection of the uterus during and after delivery, and infection that could be introduced by invasive procedures such as catheterisation, injections and infusions.

Medical Asepsis

This includes:

- General cleanliness
- Isolation of infected persons.
- Disinfection of all articles that may be contaminated, or used for more than one patient.
- Correct and frequent hand-washing by all those caring for patients.

Hand-washing Technique

- Wet the hands under running water.
- Apply soap thoroughly, and use a brush for the nails if possible.
- Rinse well.
- Dry with a clean towel. It is important to keep the nails short.

Use of Gowns, Gloves and Masks, in Medical Asepsis

Any patient who is a source of infection needs to be isolated. The type of isolation depends on the method by which the organisms may spread from person to person.

Gown

Gown protection is needed for persons in close contact with a patient who may spread infection by urine, faeces, vomit, or wound drainage. (e.g) typhoid fever, dysentery, cholera, gas gangrene.

Gloves

This is needed to protect persons coming in close contact with a patient having a communicable disease, which is air-borne. (e.g) diphtheria, sore throat, meningitis, chickenpox, whooping cough etc. In most of these cases a gown is also needed.

Gown Technique

At the entrance to the patients unit a stand should be provided on which to hang the isolation gown.

If the stand is inside the unit, the gown is hung with the contaminated side out.

- If outside the unit, it is hung clean side out.
- To put on the gown, insert your hands into the sleeves of the gown without touching the contaminated side.
- Then fasten the neck-band, which is considered clean. Fasten the belt and then carry out the work in the unit.
- After finishing, untie the belt, wash your hands and untie the neckband.
- Remove the first sleeve, remove the second sleeve by grasping it with the gown-covered hand.
- Place the gown carefully on the hook, then wash your hands again thoroughly.

Use of Gloves

Clean gloves are usually adequate in medical asepsis, but when handling a wound after surgery or the vagina during delivery or in the puerperium, sterile gloves are needed. After using the gloves, they are removed and placed into a disinfectant solution. The gloved hands may be washed under the running water before taking them off and then placed in the disinfectant solution.

Use of Masks

Clean masks should be kept in a clean area near the hand-washing facilities at the entrance of the isolation unit. Take a mask and tie it on before you enter. When leaving, wash hands, remove the mask holding the strings only, and drop it into a second container for used masks. Masks must be disinfected before being used again. Now disposable masks are available for use and throw.

Principles of Isolation technique

- The degree of isolation will depend on the type of disease.
- The patient should be isolated as long as he/she is a

source of infection. The time depends on the particular disease.

- Persons attending the patient should be limited to one or two and no visitors allowed.
- The room should have only essential furniture and be easily cleaned (Damp dusting and floor cleaning).
- Gown, apron and mask should be provided for any one entering the room. Used masks are to be dropped into disinfectant solution.
- Hands should be washed with soap and water after touching the patient. All the articles used by him should be disinfected
- Everything taken out of the room must be disinfected. Dust, excreta and discharges, waste food soiled linen and utensils, must be disposed off with care.
- For terminal disinfection, the patient is given a bath and clean clothes, and taken away from the isolation room. Then the room and everything in it is thoroughly disinfected.

Barrier Nursing

In this type of isolation, the corner of a general medical ward is suitable for patient with infections other than air-borne. (e.g) Typhoid fever, dysentery and diarrhoea. It is best if the room is screened against flies. A gown or apron and hand washing facilities are kept at the bedside. Excreta must be carefully disposed of bedpans and bed linen is disinfected. All other precautions are taken to prevent the spread of the infections.

Surgical Asepsis

This means keeping objects and areas ' sterile' free from all organisms. Surgical asepsis (Sterile technique) is used in the operating room, delivery room, in doing surgical dressings and many other invasive procedures. The nurse must thoroughly understand the principle of surgical asepsis. She must be reliable in always keeping to these principles.

She must know about the use and care of the masks, gloves and gowns, the proper technique of hand washing for surgical procedures and the sterilizing and handling of sterile equipments.

Masks, Gloves and Gowns for Surgical use

Masks

A facemask is worn when doing any sterile surgical procedures. The purpose of the mask in surgical nursing is to prevent any germs from the person' s respiratory tract from being breathed up on the wound or sterile articles.

- The mask should cover both nose and mouth of the wearer.
- It is made of two or more layers of material, either in rectangular or nosebag shape, with tapes to tie at the back of head.
- While being worn, the face piece should not be touched.
- If it becomes wet with sweat or by sneezing, it should be changed.
- Do not speak more than necessary during surgery.
- A fresh mask should be worn for each procedure.
- The mask should neither be suspended around the neck nor put into the pocket.
- After use, remove the mask, hold it by the tapes, and place it straight into antiseptic solution.
- At the end of each day, the used masks should be washed, dried, then folded with tapes outside and sterilized ready for use again.
- In some hospitals, disposable masks are worn.

loves

Surgical gloves in various sizes are made of special thin rubber so that the surgeon may not lose the sense of touch.

- In clean operations they are worn to protect the patient, but in infected cases they protect the wearer also.

- After use, gloves should be washed in cold water and then with soap and water.
- By filling the glove with water holes can be detected.
- The gloves may be wiped dry or hung on a rack and turned to dry the inside as well.
- To prepare for sterilizing, dust the gloves well both inside and out with glove powder.
- See that the roughened surface is on the outside (for better grip) then pair off the gloves.
- Turn back the cuffs 5 cm and place a small pocket of glove powder just inside the right-hand glove.
- Place the pair of gloves in a glove pocket marked with the correct size. Disposable gloves are now in use.

Gowns

Steam sterilized theatre gowns are worn by the scrubbed-up operating team, to prevent contamination of the sterile field by the contact with clothing or skin. Unsterile but clean gowns are often worn by those persons in the operating room who are not scrubbed up.

- For the surgeon and his assistant particularly, gowns should be made of close- woven material.
- For all those scrubbed up, the gowns must have sleeves, which are long enough to fit under the gloves at the wrists.
- All the gowns fasten at the back.
- An unsterile helper ties the tapes without touching the outside of the sterile gown.
- After use, gowns are soaked in cold water if blood stained, then.

  Hung to dry and sent to the laundry, or well washed in hot soapy water and ironed.
- Gowns to be sterilized must be folded and rolled up in such a way that only the inner surface is handled by the scrubbed up persons.
- They are packed in drums or bundles ready for autoclaving.

Caps, Elothing and Footwear

In the operating theatre, there must be no risk of introducing dust and dirt, especially any soil that may contain tetanus organisms. Therefore every 22 person entering must wear clean clothing, and put on clean theatre slippers or canvas shoes.

- These must be removed on leaving the theatre.
- The hair must be completely covered by means of a clean theatre cap.

Surgical Hand-Scrub

In all surgical work it is important to keep the hands and nails clean. Nails must be cut or filed very short.

- The surgical hand scrub is necessary for the surgeons and those assisting at an operation, and for sterile procedures.
- It must be realized that hands can never be made sterile except by wearing sterile gloves.

Requirements

- Running water.
- Antiseptic soap or soap solution.
- Sterile nail brush
- Sterile towel.

Method

- Wear a clean cap and then a clean mask.
- Note the time, the procedure should take 10 minutes.
- Wet the hands up to the elbows under the running water.
- Apply soap to make a good lather, and look it into the hands and arms, adding small amounts of water but not enough to remove the lather.
- After 30 seconds, rinse thoroughly.
- Apply more soap and this time uses the brush. Pay special attention to the nails, fingertips and between fingers. Add more water in small amounts frequently but keep the lather, with more soap also. After the

nails, fingers and hand, work up the arm, scrubbing gently with circular motions and following at the elbow. Repeat for the other arm.

- Rinse the arms and other hands with forearms held up so that water does not run down from the elbows to the hands.
- Dry on a sterile towel, starting with the hands and moving upwards.

Wearing Sterile Gowns and Gloves

- Take hold of the gown at arms length with your scrubbed up hands, unroll, and slip arms into the smaller, asking a helper to the tapes at the back. Both you and the helper must be very careful not to touch the outside of the gown.
- Dust your hands with sterile powder, and put on the gloves. Hold the first glove by the turned back cuff, and slip it on.
  Next insert the gloved fingers under the cuff of the second glove and slip it on. The cuff of each glove is then unfolded and pulled completely over the sleeve end of the gown. These must be no gap at the wrist, and the nurse must not touch the bare skin nor inside of glove or gown when scrubbed up.
- The first scrubbed up person may help others by holding the sterile gloves for them to slip in their hands. When scrubbed up, the nurse must remember to touch only sterile things. The instrument table and whole field of operation is draped with large sterile clothes and towels. Helpers who are not scrubbed up may help to bring sterile suppliers to the tables, keeping to the outside and using ' Cheatle forceps'.

Handling of Sterile Articles

- Always wear a mask when handling sterile articles.
- Sterilized articles must be kept in sterile containers or on sterile towels, and kept covered till used. Never allow contact of unsterile with sterile articles.

- Make sure there is no dampness, as this could make the things unsterile.
- Never allow any unsterile article including the arms and hands to pass a sterile field.
- Never touch the inside of a package or container with your fingers. Use the cheatle forceps.
- To pull a cork from a bottle of sterile fluid, take care not to contaminate the inner part neither of the cork nor inside the rim of the bottle. Replace it carefully.
- When lifting a cover from a sterile container bring it down with the inner side up and then replace it without delay. 8. To carry a sterile bowl or other container, hold it with your hands underneath, and do not touch the rim.

Rules for use of Eheatle Forceps

- The sterile jar holding the forceps must be cleaned, re-sterilized and filled with fresh antiseptic lotion daily. The cheatle forceps should be cleaned and autoclaved or boiled.
- When in use, keep the forceps at elbow level and pointed downwards because if you lift it upwards the solution may run on to your hand and then back to the forceps, making it unsterile.
- Put the forceps back into the jar immediately after use. Replace carefully without touching the rim of the jar.

  If the forceps becomes contaminated, it must be re-sterilized before being put back into the jar.

Cross Infection

Cross infection is the process of transmission of infection from one person to another person through the health care provider by using improper aseptic technique in the hospital and in the environment.

Disinfection and Methods

Disinfection is the process of killing the pathogenic or

disease producing microorganism but not usually bacterial spores. Disinfectant is germicide an agent which kills pathogenic or disease producing microorganisms but not usually bacterial spores. Eg. phenol and Lysol.

A deodorant is an agent, which suppresses bad odours. Eg. Lime, bleaching powder Detergent is a surface cleansing agent, which acts by lowering surface tension. Eg soap. Antiseptic is an agent which prevents the growth of microorganisms. Eg alcohol. Sterilization is a destruction of microorganisms and their spores.

Types of Disinfection

Concurrent Disinfection

This is disinfection of infectious material (eg stools, urine contaminated linen) through out the course of an illness. This procedure checks or prevents the dissemination or further spread of the disease agent.

Terminal Disinfection

This is disinfection that is undertaken at the termination of an illness. (eg. After recovery or death of the patient).

Prohylactic Disinfection

Boiling of water, pasteurisation of milk, washing hands with soap and water are examples. Sterilisation: It is one of the methods of disinfections which is stated above.

Methods of Disinfection

- *Natural:* Sunlight and air
- *Physical:* Dry heat, moist heat and radiation
- *Chemical:* Liquids, solids and gases.

PREPARING ARTICLES FOR DISINFECTION (STERILIZATION)

A convenient method often used is to prepare sets of the instrument, swabs, sponges, dressings, towels and the surfaces needed for each type of operation or sterile procedures.

- These sets are packed into drums, bundles or on trays, labeled and kept ready for sterilising.
- The articles should be carefully arranged so that those needed first are on top. 26
- They must be loosely packed for steam to penetrate.
- Drums or bins must have the perforations opened. 5. Bundles should have a double wrapper of close-woven cloth, or of paper.

Dressings

Swabs and sponges are usually made of several thickness of surgical gauze. Raw edges must be folded to the desired size to prepare gauze. Sponges used for abdominal surgery need to be large, stitched around the edge and a piece of tape sewed to one corner. When an artery forceps is clipped into the end of the tape, there is no risk of the sponge being left inside the abdomen.

Packing Gauze

It is made in various sizes. Use gauze four times the width of the desired packing. Fold the edges so that they meet in the middle and again fold down the centre, and roll.

Cotton Balls

It is prepared in various ways. Cotton balls of various sizes are prepared by rolling between the palms. Some may be needed for intestinal surgery, and for this the cotton ball must be covered with gauze and tied. This type of ball is grasped with a long handed forceps.

Instruments

After use, surgical instruments should be washed first in cold water then in warm water with a detergent. Use a brush to clean well especially between the teeth of artery forceps and clamps.

To be properly sterilized, there should be no dried blood or discharge. Rinse in clean water, then boil for 5 minutes and dry well.

Sharp instruments, knives and needles should be dealt with separately, taking care to avoid cuts and puncture wounds.

Glass Syringes and Metal Needles

After use, draw up some water into the glass syringe and push enough through each metal needle to make sure they are not blocked. Infected glass syringes (used for withdrawing blood or pus) should be washed immediately in cold disinfectant solution. 27 Next wash the syringes and needles in warm soapy water, using a bottle brush for the barrel.

Rinse in clean water. Take care not to get barrels and plungers mixed, but keep them always paired together. Needles should be examined carefully for sharpness. Take care not to prick your finger as infection may be transmitted in this way.

Rubber Tubing

After use tubes should be cleaned with cold water, then with hot soapy water and then rinsed. The inside must be thoroughly cleaned. Then it is boiled, and hung over. Rubber catheters should be cleaned by running cold water through from both ends. Wash and rinse in cold water, then dry, with a towel or by hanging up. Autoclave the catheters before use.

DISINFECTING METHODS (STERILISATION- PHYSICAL)

Dry heat

- Sterilizing of glassware including syringes is often done in a hot air oven at 1600c for one hour.
- Spores as well as organisms are killed. Rubber articles will not withstand this heat.
- This method is not efficient where heat has to penetrate as in dressings, towels and gowns.

Moist heat: Autoclaving (Steam under Pressure)

- This is a reliable method and may be used for most articles.

- The autoclave is a chamber with an outer jacket and a lid or door, which can be firmly clamped.
- Steam, is generated by heating water in a boiler or in the outer jacket.
- Air is evacuated from the chamber by displacement.
- Then the steam is allowed to build up pressure, usually 15 to 20 lbs per square inches, and is kept at that pressure for 15 to 30 minutes. 28
- Then the heat is turned off and the contents of the autoclave allowed to dry out.
- They should be quite dry when removed from the autoclave.

Points to Remember

- All articles should be clean and dry before packing. Any organic matter such as blood or pus prevents penetration of steam.
- The holder in the drums must be open when placing into the autoclave and closed immediately on taking them out.
- Bundles should be neither be too large nor be too tightly packed. Steam should be able to penetrate to the centre.
- Rubber gloves cannot withstand high temperature and long sterilising. Autoclave them separately at 15 lbs pressure for 15 minutes.
- To autoclave bottles of fluid, loosen the screw cops, evacuate the steam slowly.

Boiling

- This method is suitable for enamel, metal, glass and rubber ware.
- Bowl sterilizers are used for larger articles and instrument sterilizers for smaller articles.

Points to Remember

- See that the articles are quiet clean and completely immersed in clean water.

- When the water boils, start timing. If more articles are added, the sterilizing time must begin again.
- Boil for 5 minutes. iv. Boiling will not kill spores v. Remove articles with sterile cheatle or other lifting forceps, and place them on a sterile surface.
- Chemical disinfection: This method is used for sterilising delicate instruments such as eye instruments. 29 Points to remember: i) The articles must be clean and free from pus, blood or oil. ii) They must be completely immersed in the disinfectant. iii) The disinfectant should be of certain strength, and the articles must be in contact with it for a specific period. iv) After sterilization, articles must be well rinsed in sterile water before use.

NUTRITION AND DIET THERAPY

In order to live a healthy life we need all kinds of nutrients in correct proportion. Plants need sunlight, water, soil and manure for their growth.

Like that human beings need nutrients of different kinds for their optimum growth and development and maintenance of health. The word ' nutrition' comes from the word ' nourish' and it includes all the ways in which the foodstuffs we eat are absorbed by the body for the growth and development, energy and good health.

NUTRITION AND HEALTH

When a person does not eat the right nutrients in right quantity he or she is malnourished and we call this condition as malnutrition. Malnutrition is very common among children in India. He or she is under-weight because of not having enough kind of food needed for their growth. In many parts of India 40 per cent of children is under-weight for their ages.

When an under-weight child gets measles or diarrhea or some other infection, the malnutrition gets worsened and he may die. A well-nourished child is less likely to become sick and if at all he is infected, he is able to overcome the disease condition.

Malnutrition also affects the intelligence of a child. His or her trouble may start even before birth if his mother does not have the right foods when she is pregnant. The malnourished child is slow in learning and doing. Adult people who are malnourished are not able to work optimum. Production and development of the country are slowed down because of malnutrition.

Every one needs enough right kinds of food. Here is comparison of the effects on the people of good nutrition and malnutrition.

Food and Nutrients

Food means any substance, which can be used to the body for nourishment, that is, for its growth and maintenance. Food is necessary for life.

Foods are obtained from plants of many kinds, and from birds, fish and animals. Nutrients are materials present in food: They are,

- Proteins.
- Carbohydrates
- Fats and oils.
- Vitamins.
- Minerals
- Water.

Most food contains several of these nutrients. There is no one food in nature, which contains all nutrients. We need to know different kinds of foods, what nutrients they contain and why they are important.

Functions of Food

- For growth and development, and repairing of tissues- Protein food mainly.
- To provide energy for doing work-stable foods and fats.
- To help the body to function properly and to protect from diseases- vitamins and minerals. When all these functions are fulfilled in the body, a person is in a state of good health.

Energy Yielding Food

A continual need of the body is energy. Energy foodstuffs are fuel for the body to work, like diesel is the fuel for a bus to run. The harder you work, the more energy food you need. Even at rest, the body still uses energy for breathing and for the heart beating.

While burning fuel foods for energy, heat is also produced. In cold weather one can keep oneself warm by exercising and eating more energy foods. Stable foods are cheap sources of energy.

They are the basis of our diet. They contain mostly carbohydrates and also proteins in small amount. The kind of stable food we eat depends on our food habits and also what are available. The stable food includes:

- Cereals and grains: Wheat made into bread, chappati etc, rice, jowar, maize, ragi and millets.
- Starchy vegetables: Potatoes, sweet potato and tapioca.
- Starchy fruits: Banana, jackfruit, mango etc.
- Sugar, honey and jaggery provide extra energy.

They are rich in carbohydrates foods. Fats and oils such as vanaspathi, butter, ghee, oilseeds and cooking oils are good sources of energy but they are not cheap. We should include them with each meal. Fatstores in the body are useful when more energy is needed.

Calories are the unit to measure energy. We use calories to measure how much of energy is there in certain foods. We also use calories to measure how much of energy a person needs (energy requirements).

- One gram of carbohydrate yields four calories.
- One gram of fat yields nine calories.
- One gram of protein yields four calories. Proteins are not included in energy yielding food because they are mainly used for bodybuilding. Here are some foodstuffs and the calories provided per 100 grams.

Proteins or the Body-Builders

Proteins are essential for growth, for building different

kinds of cells, tissues and organs of the human body. From this we can understand why pregnant women, nursing mothers, babies and children all need to have a lot of proteins in their diet.

Those who are injured or diseased need extra protein for repair of tissue. Everyone needs protein because our bodies are made up of living cells, which wear out and need replacing. For example, the life of red blood cells is only about 120 days. New red blood cells need to be synthesized constantly.

Food stuff	Calories
1. Cow milk	65
2. Buffalo milk	117
3. Jaggery	383
4. Honey	320
5. Sesame seeds	564
6. Groundnuts	549
7. Banana	150
8. Tapioca	159
9. Sweet potato	132
10. Potato	99
11. Wheat bread	238
12. Wheat flour	348
13. Chappati	124
14. Rice	345
15. Ragi	331
16. Maize	342
17. Bajra	360

Calorie Requirements (Energy Requirements)

- A baby below 6 months needs 120 calories per kg of body weight per day.
- A baby, 7 to 12 months age needs 100 calories/kg per day.
- A child, 1-3 years old needs about 1200 calories per day.

- A child, 4-6 years old needs about 1600 calories per day.
- A child, 7-9 years old needs about 1800 calories per day.
- A child, 10-12 years old needs about 2100 calories per day.
  An adolescent girl 13-19 years old and boy 13-15 years old needs 2300 calorie per day.
- An adolescent boy 16-19 years old needs 3000 calories per day.
- A man with moderate work needs 2800 calories per day.
- A woman with moderate work needs 2200 calories per day.
- A woman who is pregnant needs extra 300 calories per day.
- A woman who is lactating needs extra 500 calories per day.

Amino Acids

There are different types of proteins and each one is made up of different type of amino acids. There are about 20 different kinds of amino acids. When we eat a protein food, first the protein gets separated and then the protein chain is broken into amino acids.

Inside the body new proteins are synthesized by joining up the amino acids in different order according to the needs of the body. These are called body proteins. The body can make some amino acids out of others, and these are called ' nonessential amino acids'.

About 8 amino acids cannot be made by the body and must be taken in our food. They are called the ' essential amino acids'. The protein in milk and eggs provide all these essential amino acids and these are the best bodybuilding food. Other animal proteins (meat and fish) are also good body-builders. Vegetarians and people who cannot afford to have animal proteins can get enough essential amino acids by mixing and including more variety of plant protein food. Many amino acids in our food are not useful for bodybuilding and so are used as fuel for energy. Those who do not get enough of the essential amino acids in their diet become malnourished. However, it is often possible to get the amino acids we need by eating two kinds of plant proteins at one time. For example, proteins in rice are short of two essential amino acids, but pulses are rich sources of these amino acids.

Therefore mixing pulses with rice makes a more nutritious diet. In a similar way, soy flour (from soyabeans) can be mixed with wheat flour to make nutritious roti or chappaties. A mixed cereal diet is better than just one kind of cereal. A poor family at least can cook some dark green leafy vegetables to eat with the stable food and this will help in providing some proteins.

Functions, Sources and Daily Requirements of Proteins, Carbohydrates and Fats

Proteins: Functions

- For body growth (body-building)
- Repair of worn out tissues and healing of wounds.
- For the blood, to make hemoglobin and blood proteins.
- For making enzymes and hormones.
- For secretion of mother' s milk.
- For the development of antibodies to protect against infections.
- May be used for energy.

Sources

Animal proteins (best for body-building): Milk, curds, cheese, egg, fish and meat. Vegetable proteins: Groundnuts and soya beans are the best sources of proteins. Cereals, pulses (dhal and grams) legumes (peas and beans) oil seeds.

Deficiency

The effects of protein deficiency include the following:

- In pregnant woman the baby may be stillborn or premature

- In infants and early childhood: Stunted growth and mental retardation, kwashiorkor.
- In adults, weakness, anemia, thin muscles, diarrhoea, recurrent infections, delay in wound healing, edema, ascites and liver cirrhosis.

Kwashiorkor

It is also called wet malnutrition. It is caused by not eating enough protein. A child with kwashiorkor may look fat, but he has edema. He has swollen feet, hands and face. When we press the swollen parts, your finger makes a depression or dimple because there is fluid accumulation under the skin. He may be over-weight because of the edema, but when the edema goes, his weight will fall down.

Even with edema, the upper arms will be thin, and the arm circumference is low. The child with kwashiorkor also has sores with peeling skin, his hair loses its natural colour, and he is likely to have diarrhoea. He is unhappy, and not active like other children of his age. Kwashiorkor is the most common in children between 1 - 2 years.

Often it first appears in a child following a diarrhoeal or measles infection. Children with kwashiorkor need extra food, especially foods rich in protein. If possible give eggs, chicken meat and fish. Poor families who cannot afford these may prefer soya beans and groundnuts which are good and cheap sources of protein. Soya beans need to be soaked well before being cooked, or made into flour and mixed with other flour to make porridge. If a child with kwashiorkor is not able to take feeds, he must be tube-fed, with high protein - calorie liquid foods, about 150 ml per kg per day.

Carbohydrates Functions

- Provide energy for work
- Produce heat
- Help in metabolism of fats and proteins.
- Cellulose (fibre) a type of carbohydrate prevents, constipation Sources: Cereals: rice, wheat, jowar, maize, rag

- Sugars: White sugar, jaggery, honey, glucose. Root vegetables: Potato, sweet potato, tapioco. Fruits: Banana, jackfruit, mango etc. Recommended dietary allowance (RDA) is 1 gram of protein per kg of body weight.

Deficiency

Marasmus' is a deficiency condition in which the child is small, very thin, with no fat under his skin and with muscles 41 wasting.

His face is so thin that he looks like a little old man. He is only about half the weight that he should be for his age. His midarm circumference is much less than 14 cm. He may have chronic diarrhea. The cause of marasmus may be

- Loss of mother
- Lack of breast milk.
- Bottle feeds
- Recurrent diarrhoea, The child with marasmus needs sufficient food.

Fats Functions

- It acts as a concentrated energy source.
- It helps in absorption of fat soluble vitamins (vitamins A, D, E and K).
- It makes food tasty and satisfies the appetite.
- Fat stored in the body protects one from cold and is a reserve source of energy. 5. It gives energy and heat to the body.

Sources

- Sesame oil.
- Sunflower seed oil
- Cottonseed oil
- Soyabean oil.

Other sources

- Groundnut oils, coconut oil, mustard oil.
- Vanaspati, butter, ghee, cheese, milk, curds, fish and fatty meat.

- Deficiency: Deficiency of fats leads to dry skin (toad skin).

Vitamins and minerals-protective foods

Vitamins and minerals are micronutrients, as very small amounts of vitamins and minerals are needed every day to keep the body in good health. Many foods contain vitamins and minerals as well as proteins, carbohydrates and Fats. Vitamins and minerals regulate the body functions.

Vitamins

Vita' means life. Deficiency of vitamins results in ill-health and even death. There are two groups: a. Fat- soluble vitamins: A, D, E, and K. b. Water soluble Vitamins: B and C. Vitamin A: Vitamin A is needed in the body for

- Healthy eyes.
- Healthy skin and mucous membrane.

Recommended dietary allowance (RDA): A daily requirement of vitamin A is 800 micrograms. Too much is harmful.

Sources: Fish liver oil, egg, butter, ghee and milk are rich sources of vitamin A. In plants there is a substance called carotene or provitamin A, which can be made into Vitamin A in the body. Sources of carotene are dark green leafy vegetables and yellow fruits and vegetables such as carrot, papaya, ripe mango, yellow pumpkin.

Deficiency: If a person does not have enough Vitamin A, he gets night blindness, then dry eye, and may become blind. Vitamin D: Uses It helps in absorption of calcium and phosphorus to build bones and teeth.

Sources

- Sunlight is the cheapest source. Vitamin D formed in the skin by the action of ultra-violet rays in sunlight.
- Fish liver oil.
- Butter, ghee, groundnut oil and egg yoke. Recommended dietary allowance (RDA): 400 internal units. Deficiency: Deficiency leads to rickets

Vitamin E: Vitamin E is essential for normal reproduction.

Deficiency: Deficiency may lead to infertility.

Vitamin K: Vitamin K is the necessary for blood clotting. It is used in prevention and treatment of hemorrhage. Sources:

- Dark green leaves of all kinds, pulses, cereals and fruits.
- It is also produced by bacteria in the small intestine. Sprouted grains.
- Dairy products. Recommended dietary allowance (RDA): 60 micrograms per day.

Deficiency: Deficiency leads to bleeding disorders.

Water Soluble Vitamins

Vitamin B and C Vitamin B1 or Thiamine: Vitamin B1 or Thiamine is necessary for carbohydrate metabolism and conduction of nerve impulses Sources: Dried fruits, yeasts, unpolished rice, whole wheat flour, whole cereals and pulses, nuts and oils seeds, liver and green leafy vegetables. Recommended dietary allowance (RDA):

- Milligram per day Deficiency: This is common where people eat a lot of raw polished rice, as in parts of Andhra Pradesh. Early symptoms are
- Loss of appetite
- Tingling hands and feet, or numbness.
- Restlessness and general weakness.
- Breathlessness due to heart enlargements. 5. Leads to loss of memory and nervous disorder. If thiamine deficiency continuous, it results in the disease called beri-ber
  - There are two forms of beri-ber
  - In the wet type, there is edema or swelling all over the body. In the dry type, there is paralysis. Infantile beri-beri can result in early sudden death due to enlarged heart.In deficiency of thiamine, there is usually also deficiency of riboflavin and nicotinic acid. Therefore vitamin B Complex is needed in its treatment, as well as extra thiamine.

Riboflavin: Vitamin B2

Riboflavin is necessary for

- Metabolism of carbohydrates, fats and amino acids.
- Healthy eyes and mouth. Sources: Dried yeast, whole cereals, pulses and dark green leafy vegetables, milk and eggs, and liver. Recommended dietary allowance (RDA): 1 - 2 milligram per day.

Deficiency

Signs of this are

- Angular stomatitis-sore white patches at the corners of the mouth.
- Glossitis-swollen sore tongue.
- Redness and burning feeling in the eyes.
- dermatitis -skin lesions.

Nicotinic acid

Nicotinic acid (Niacin) is needed for

- Carbohydrate metabolism along with thiamine and riboflavin
- Healthy skin and mucous membrane
- Healthy nervous system.

Sources

Dried yeast, whole cereals, groundnuts and pulses, liver, meat and fish. Recommended dietary allowance (RDA): 15 milligram per day

Deficiency

Deficiency leads to a disease called pellagra. The signs are

- Sore tongue, with teeth marks made by the teeth.
- Dermatitis- dark patches on exposed parts of the skin. Diarrhoea
- Dementia- loss of memory. Advanced stage of pellagra usually ends in death. For both Riboflavin and Nicotinic acid deficiency, vitamin B complex is given.

Folic Acid

Folic acid is needed for synthesis of red blood cells and in the formation of new tissues.

Sources: Dried yeast, liver and egg, cereals, pulses, nuts and oil seeds, dark green leafy vegetables and other vegetables. Recommended dietary allowance (RDA): 180 microgram per day. For pregnant and lactating women need 300 micrograms per day

Vitamin B12: (cobalamin)

Vitamin 12 is also needed for synthesis of red blood cells.

Sources: Milk, eggs and meat especially liver. Recommended dietary allowance (RDA): 2 microgram per day. Deficiency: B12 deficiency leads to pernicious anemia.

Vitamin B6: (pyridoxine)

Vitamin B6 is necessary for carbohydrate and fat metabolism.

Vitamin C is necessary to

- Keep body tissues intact
- Help in repair of tissues.
- Protect the body against infections.
- Absorb iron. Sources: Drumsticks and their leaves, amla (nellikai), bitter gourd guava, sprouted grain, citrus fruits such as oranges and lemons, papaya, tomato. The vitamin is very easily destroyed by heat, light and drying. Recommended dietary allowance (RDA): 30-50 mg, and for lactating women 80 mg. Deficiency: This results in scurvy. It is found in infants who are given inadequate feeds and those who do not take enough fresh fruits and vegetables containing vitamin C.

Signs and Symptoms of scurvy are

- Spongy, bleeding gums and loose teeth.
- Bleeding under the skin and into various tissues.
- Pain and swelling in the joints.
- Slow healing of wounds, or breakdown of old wound scars. Treatment is with ascorbic acid (vitamin C) tablets or multivitamin tablets, and advice about diet. Infants who are not breast fed need vitamin C, and

given in the form of fruit juice or vegetable juice. Those recovering from illness such as diarrhoea, or from wounds, need more of this vitamin.

Minerals

Plants absorb minerals in the soil and water. Animals and human beings eat plants. Therefore we get minerals from three sources: Water, plants and animals.

Calcium

This mineral is present in large amounts in bones and teeth. Therefore extra calcium is needed for pregnant and nursing mothers and growing children.

Functions

Calcium is necessary for

- Formation of bones and teeth
- Clotting of blood.
- Strength of capillary walls.
- Contraction of heart muscle and skeletal muscles.
- Normal functioning of nerves. Calcium needs to be in correct proportion with phosphorus. Vitamins D and C are also needed for calcium absorption and utilization.

Sources: Milk is an important source. Other sources are ragi, bajra, sesame seeds, wheat, small dried fish and seafood. Recommended dietary allowance (RDA): 1200 mg per day

Calcium Deficiency

This may result in

- Stunted growth in children.
- Rickets (Calcium and vitamin D deficiency)
- Tetany-nervousness, muscles twitching and spasms.

Osteoporosis - Brittle Bones so that Fractures Occur with Minor Accidents.

Interference with Blood Clotting. Phosphorus

Phosphorus is needed

- With calcium to form bones and teeth.
- For brain and nerves formation.
- For carbohydrates and fat metabolism.
- For development of all types of cells in the body.

Sources

Most food contain phosphorus, especially milk, meat, fish, eggs, nuts grains and green leaves. Recommended dietary allowance (RDA): 1200 mg per day.

Iron

Iron is necessary for synthesis of hemoglobin in the blood. Pregnant women need extra iron for the development of fetal blood. Iron is lost in menstruation and whenever there is bleeding deficiency of iron causes anemia. Vitamin C helps in the absorption of iron. Sources: Ragi, bajra, sesame seeds, jaggery, dark green leafy vegetables, gram and dhal, liver, meat and eggs. Recommended dietary allowance (RDA): 25 mg for men and 35 mg for women per day.

Deficiency

Insufficiency of iron in the diet is a common cause of anemia. Those who lack iron look pale, have difficulties in breathing and get easily tired. Children who are anemia are often sick. Normally the iron in our bodies is reused and hence we need little extra iron from our diet. In the following circumstances iron is lost and anemia develops.

- Bleeding of any kind, excess bleeding during menstruation, bleeding piles and dysentery.
- Disease such as malaria and hookworm, where blood is destroyed.
- In pregnancy because the fetus takes iron from the mother. Growing children need extra iron to synthesis blood, and anemia is common especially after the age of 3 or 4 months when the iron stored in the liver is depleted. There is very little iron in milk, and other iron rich foods must be given to these young children.

Iodine

Iodine is needed for the normal functioning of the thyroid gland.

Sources

- Sea fish, vegetables grown near the seawater.
- Iodized salt should be used. Recommended dietary allowance (RDA): 150 mg per day.

Deficiency: In places far from the sea there is deficiency of iodine in water and food (Himalayan belt). In many people, especially girls, the thyroid gland enlarges leading to a condition called goiter.

- Goitre is an endemic disease.
- During pregnancy iodine deficiency causes cretinism in the baby.
- Goitre may be prevented and also cured by the regular use of iodized salt in the diet of people who live in areas of iodine deficiency.
- Under the National Goitre Control Programme (NGCP), iodized salt is supplied freely in endemic goitre area, with the help of UNICEF.

Water

Water is a basic requirement. More than 60per cent of the human body weight is due to water.

Distribution of Water

Water is distributed in three compartments

- Intercellular (50per cent of the body weight)
- Interstitial (15per cent of the body weight)
- Blood (5 per cent of the body weight)

Sources: Sources of Water are Drinking Water, Food and a Small Quantity is Formed as a Result of Metabolism (800ml). Functions

- Essential constituents of many vital body fluids (blood, lymph, CSF)

  Assists in the regulation of the body temperature.

- Helps in the transport of nutrition' s within the body
- building and repair of the body tissues. 5. Utilised in body processes. Eg. Digestion, absorption, elimination 6. Besides body needs water for bathing, washing and other activities.

Water loss: Water is lost through urine, sweat, expired air, in the faeces and lactating women through the milk Requirement for a normal healthy person needs 6 glasses of water. (1 ml per calorie of food) Pathologic effect of excessive water loss occurs in severe diarrhoea, resulting in dehydration. Water retention (kidney failure results in enema

BALANCED DIET

The balanced diet is the basis of good nutrition, and necessary for every member of the family. Balanced diet means is the diet, which contains all the nutrients in the right proportion necessary for our body to be healthy and strong. The amount will vary according to age and other factors. Most people in India eat an ill-balanced diet of mainly rice or chappaties and very little of other foods. To be healthy everyone needs to eat a balanced diet comprising of different nutrients in correct proportion.

We Should Select Foodstuff From Each of the Following Groups

- Stable foods: Rice, wheat, millets, starchy vegetables or fruits like banana. These foods provide calories for energy and some proteins. Remember that eating a mixture of stable foods at each meal gives better protein value.

Extra Protein Foods

- Pulses such as dhal and beans, nuts, and dark green leaves
- Milk and milk products, eggs, meat and fish.

Protective Foods,

- Containing a lot of vitamins and minerals including:

- Vegetables, dark green leafy vegetables
- Yellow fruits, citrus fruits and others.

Fats and Sugars for Extra Energy

- A little fat or oil used in cooking or taken with each meal. ii) Jaggery, sugar and honey, for extra calories when needed. Note that dark green leafy vegetables are in the group of protective foods and in the extra protein group. They are the most valuable cheap food containing a lot of nutrients. They may even be collected in the fields in some places, or grown in kitchen gardens.

Vulnerable Groups

Some groups in our communities are more likely to lack a balanced diet and to suffer from malnutrition. They are called the vulnerable groups. Vulnerable groups who need special attention with regard to nutrition are as follows.

- Infants: Birth to one year.
- Toddlers: 1-3 years
- Pre school children: 4 or 5 years.

  School children and adolescents. 5. Pregnant and lactating mothers. 6. Old people. 7. The sick, those need a modified diet.

Infants

Breast milk is the best food for infants. It is not sufficient after six months. From fourth month onward a child can start having porridge (conjee) made with milk, dhal rice, mashed potatoes and green leaves etc. Children 1-3 years need about 1200 calories per day.

Daily requirements	Remarks.
stable foods 150 gm (at least two kinds including ragi or bajra)	Serve three times per day.
milk 200 ml * egg, fish or meat 30 gm pulses. 40 gm dark green leafy vegetables 50gm	* Instead of this, vegetarians need extra 100 ml milk and 10 gm pulses.
other vegetables 30 gm fruits 50 gm	Preferably carrot, pumpkin or other sources of carotene.
sugar or jaggery 30 gm oil 20 gm	Jaggery provides extra iron and costs less.

Daily Menu for Children of 1 - 3 Years

6 a.m	100-150 ml milk with sugar or jaggery
8 a.m	Porridge 100 ml
10 a.m	Fresh fruit (100 gm) such as banana, guava, tomato, papaya or mango.
12 noon	75-100 gm well-cooked rice or other stable food. One boiled and mashed egg or fish or meat or 2 spoons well-cooked and mashed dhal. 3-4 spoons boiled dark green leafy vegetable 1 spoon ghee or oil, added and well mixed in the food while hot.
3 p.m	Pulse such as Bengal gram, 1 handful. Milk with sugar or jaggary.
7.30 p.m	Meal similar to 12-noon meal.

Children 4-6 Years

Children 4-6 years need about 1500 calories per day, with requirements as follows.

- Stable foods (two) 200 gm
- Milk 200 ml
- Egg, fish and meat -for vegetarians give extra milk and pulses. 30 gm
- Pulses. 50 gm
- Dark green leafy vegetables - Give vegetable salad 3 times per week. 75 gm
- Other vegetables 50 gm
- Fruit 50 gm
- Sugar and jaggery 40 gm
- Oil. 25 gm

School Children

School children need to have a good breakfast and to have balanced midday meal at school. In the evening they again need to have a well-balanced meal with the family.They need one or two snacks during the day. If a midday meal is not provided at school, the child should be given a packed meal to take to school.

A packed meal from home could include chappaties with thick dhal, boiled beans or groundnut, butter, and one fresh fruit.

Pregnant and Lactating Women Need About as Follows

Foodstuffs	Pregnant Woman		Lactating Woman	
	Veg. gm/day	Non veg gm/day	Veg gm/day	Non veg gm/day
Stable Food Cereals in 3 months (include ragi or bajra)	400	400	500	475
Extra Proteins				
Pulses- 2 servings	80	50	100	50
Nuts	60	40	100	80
Meat, Fish or egg	--	85	--	100
milk and curds	600	450	800	650
Protective Foods				
Dark green leafy vegetables	100	100	100	100
Other vegetables	75	75	75	75
Fruits.	60	60	60	60
Extra Energy foods				
Fats and oils	35	35	45	45
sugar and jaggery	30	30	30	30

If a pregnant or lactating woman is pure vegetarian or cannot afford to have milk, she should be encouraged to

- Increase the pulses in her diet.
- Eat a handful of groundnuts daily.
- Drink milk made from ragi, malt, groundnuts or soybeans.

Old People

Old people need less calories than others, and eat only a small amount at a time. The diet should include some protein and protective foods every day.

Foodstuffs	Veg gm/day	Non veg gm/day
Cereals in 3 servings (including ragi or bajra)	300	300
Pulses	70	55
Groundnuts and sesame seeds	50	30
Milk	300	200
Meat, fish and eggs.	----	30
Dark green leafy vegetables	100	100
Other vegetables	50	50
Fats and oils	20	20
Sugar and jaggery	20	20

Educate the community about balanced diet especially for vulnerable groups (Mothers and children) as follows:

- If children under 5 years do not have a balanced diet

they easily get sick and may die or grow up weak in body and mind.

- If a pregnant woman does not have a balanced diet (enough of the right kinds of foods every day) her baby when born is likely to be small and weak. Also she will not have sufficient breast milk.
- Pregnant and nursing woman need to eat more than they eat normally, with extra protein and protective foods for health of themselves and the babies they are nourishing.
- The nursing mother should continue to have extra nutritious foods, and include green and yellow vegetables daily. She also needs to drink more including milk or milk substitutes.
- Breast milk is the ideal food for babies, and should be continued as long as possible. Other foods need to be given in addition from the 4th month.
- Make sure that all infants receive a balanced diet that with something from each of the food groups. At one year a child should be having all kinds of solid food plus breastfeeding or about four cups of milk.
- Children need to have regular balanced meals, and should not be made to wait long or to skip meals. They need three good meals a day and extra snacks. For snacks give fruits, pulses and nuts.
- Foods given to children should be
  - Well prepared in clean conditions.
  - Not highly spiced, nor with a lot of sugar.
  - Well-cooked, and served fresh.
- Rapidly growing school children need a good balanced diet with extra body-building and protective foods.
- Adolescents need plenty of energy foods in addition to foods containing other nutrients. Adolescent girls need extra dark green leafy vegetables for iron to make hemoglobin.

Dietary Needs of Patients

When a person has some health problem, diet is often

more important than medicine. When a person is ill and if the correct diet is given, he or she will recover quickly. If sickness is prolonged (chronic illness), diet is important in keeping up the strength. The nurse should know what to advise about modified diets for persons who are sick and those with special health problems. In the home, the family will need the nurse' s help in the selection and preparation of foods for persons with special dietary needs.

TYPES OF DIETS

Full Diet

For the patients who are well, a well-balanced full diet should be served, either vegetarian or non-vegetarian as desired. Patients with tuberculosis should be encouraged to take a full diet to gain weight.

Liquid Diet

This is needed for patients with high fever, and those who are unable to take solid food. When no solid food is taken, a total of at least 2000 ml per day of liquids will be needed for an adult patient. If the patient can swallow only a little at a time, liquids should be given every few minutes. Milk is the basis of a good liquid diet, and it may be enriched by adding egg, ragi, skimmed milk powder, or cream.

Different flavours may be added to milk such as cocoa, coffee or fruit also sugar or glucose. Well-cooked and strained cereal conjee may be allowed, and ghee or vegetable oil any be added for more calories. Strained dhal water, or soups made with meat or vegetables may be given. Fruit juices, coconut water and barley water are other liquids that may be given.

Soft, Semi-Solid and Light Diets

These are between liquid and full diet. The reason may be that the patient is unable to masticate, or has difficulty in swallowing. A patient with moderate fever and one, who is recovering from an illness or surgery, should be given light diet. The diet should be equally nutritious and balanced as a full diet, but more easily digested and with less roughage. Avoid oily, fried foods and greasy sweets.

Cook well by a simple method using little or no spices and condiments. Foods may be minced or mashed to make them soft. Make sure that highly nutritious foods are included, such as green leafy vegetables, dhal, curds, eggs, meat and fish for non-vegetarian light diet.

Bland Diet

This is a soft and easily digestible diet without spices, condiments, coffee or any other stimulant. It is often ordered in gastro intestinal disorders.

High Protein Diet

This is ordered for patients with burns, protein deficiency disease, preeclampsia, anemia and in chronic kidney disease. About one litre of milk should be taken each day, and extra protein can be supplied by adding skimmed milk powder or egg to the milk. Mixed protein-rich foods like groundnuts, grams and dhal may be ground and cooked with the stable cereal. Non-vegetarians may have fish and meat.

Low Protein Diet

This is ordered for patients with acute nephritis. It is continued as long as there is too much urea in the blood. Easily digested carbohydrate foods with a little ghee or butter may be allowed, and boiled sweets. At first the diet may be only fruit juice with glucose. A little milk may be allowed later.

Salt- Free Diet or low Salt Diet

This is given to control edema, because sodium is closely connected with fluid retention in the body. Edema occurs in the following conditions. Acute nephritis and subacute nephritis, anemia, congestive cardiac failure, preeclampsia (in pregnancy). For a salt-free diet no salt is allowed in the preparation of foods.

Sugar or limejuice may be added for giving taste. Dried fish should be avoided as it contains more salt.

Low-fat Diet

Fats are digested with the help of bile. In diseases affecting the liver, bile is not produced in sufficient quantity. Also in gall bladder disease the bile may not reach the duodenum. Therefore in liver and gall bladder diseases a low-fat or fatfree diet may be ordered. Skimmed milk is allowed. Glucose, sugar or jaggery, rice, bread, dhal, greens and vegetables and fruits are allowed provided that no fat is used in cooking.

Low Residual Diet

This is a diet without roughage or anything that stimulates the bowel. This is ordered in cases such as colitis, colostomy, and may be ordered for a few days after perineal suturing. Arrowroot, milk and eggs, tea, toast, strained fruit juice is allowed. Vegetables and fruits are softened and filtered through a sieve. Avoid rough cereals, green vegetables, dhal, peas, beans etc.

Low Calorie Diet

This is ordered for patients with obesity or heart conditions in which it is necessary to reduce the body weight. When calories are reduced in the diet, the body takes and uses the stored fat. A low calorie diet may also be ordered for a patient with diabetes. a. Sugar and jaggery are not allowed. A substitute sweetener can be used in coffee and tea etc. b. Only a little fat or oil may be used in cooking. c.

Cereals are allowed only in very small quantities. d. Potatoes and yams are not allowed, but other vegetables and greens may be eaten in greater quantities. e. Fruits are allowed but not more than one 100 gm a day. f. Protein foods including milk, curds, eggs, cheese, fish, chicken, meat (without fat), dhal etc may be given liberally.

Diet in Special Conditions (Diet Therapy)

Peptic Ulcer

This is a chronic ulcer in the inner lining of the stomach or duodenum. The gastric juice contains hydrochloric acid, which erodes the mucus lining and thus prevents healing of the ulcer. A person who has a peptic ulcer complains of pain in the upper abdomen, which gets worse two or three hours after eating.

The pain is worse at night and if a meal is missed. At first, there may be only indigestion and heartburn. Later, besides pain, there may be vomiting with blood. The motion may be black like tar, due to internal bleeding. The ulcer may get deeper and cause a hole in the wall of the stomach or duodenum, leading to perforation and peritonitis. Bleeding and peritonitis cause death if the condition is not treated immediately. Peptic ulcer should be prevented by diet and healthy eating habits. For those with peptic ulcer, advise as follows:

- Have meals at regular times. A bland diet is needed.
- Avoid too much spicy, greasy and heavy meals.
- Avoid smoking and alcoholic drinks.
- Advise to avoid tension and anger.
- Avoid coffee and tea.

Menu for Peptic Ulcer Patients

6 a.m: Milk two cups. 8 a.m: Bread two slices, and butter 2 teaspoon, boiled eggs, or cheese two slices, or ground nuts 2 tablespoons and milk two cups. 10 a.m: Milk with sugar two cups. 12 noon: Rice or bread, mashed dhal one cup-minced meat or fish, or cheese or groundnut as above. Boiled potato, and mashed leafy vegetables one cup. Milk pudding cup. 2 p.m: Milk one cup. 4. p.m: Milk with sugar one cup, and two biscuits. 6 p.m: Milk with sugar two cups. 8.p.m: Similar to 12 noon meal. 10 p.m: Milk one cup.

Renal Disease

The special diet for kidney diseases nephritis has already been mentioned (see low protein diet). For urinary tract infections and renal stones, give plenty of fluids. If there is no fever, a bland, well-balanced diet may be given.

Diabetes Mellitus

In this disease, there is more glucose level in the blood

than normal and some glucose is excreted in the urine. It is due to deficiency or absence of insulin, a hormone produced by the Islets of Langerhans of pancreas. It is common among rice-eaters and usually starts at about 40 years of age. Diet in this disease must be strictly regulated according to the amount of glucose found in urine and the amount of insulin ordered by the doctor.

When an injection of insulin has been given food also has to be given and the doctor' s instructions must be strictly followed. The patient must be helped to understand the causes of coma.

The nurse must advise the patient to prevent forbidden foods such as sweets and sweetened coffee. A diet, outlined in low calorie diet is usually ordered.

Hypertension: (High Blood Pressure)

This is a common condition in middle age, especially in obese people. It can lead to complications such as heart disease, kidney disease and stroke.

To Prevent and Treat Hypertension

- Over-weight people should lose weight (see low calorie diet)
- Low-fat, salt-free diet is needed.
- Coffee and other stimulants should be avoided.
- Get the person to relax and avoid tension.

Heart Disease

Heart diseases are more common among older people, especially those who are fat, those who smoke, and those with hypertension. Diet is important in the treatment and care of those with heart problems. The diet should be low in cholesterol and rich in essential fatty acids. Those who are over-weight should have less calories. They should have little or no salt.

Jaundice

Jaundice is the symptom of liver disorders. Liver is the

important organ for fat digestion. Hence fat free and carbho hydrate rich diet should be prescribed for these patients.

PREPARATION OF SPECIAL DIETS

- *Fruit juice*: Use a fruit squeezer to extract the juice of a lemon or lime. Strain the juice through a seive. Add an equal quantity of drinking water and sugar or glucose to sweeten.
- *Barley water*: Wash the barley. Add two tablespoons to a little of cold water. Bring to boil and simmer gently for one hour. Strain and add limejuice and sugar for taste.
- *Tea*: Boil some clean water. Pour a little boiling water into the teapot to warm it, and pour this away. Put tea-leaves into the teapot (about 1 teaspoonful per person) and pour on boiling water, cover the teapot and leave it to stand for about 2 minutes before serving. Add a little milk and sugar or limejuice.
- *Egg flip*: Beat up an egg and then add to it a tumbler full of warm milk slowly, beating all the time. Add a little sugar or glucose if desired.
- *Boiled egg*: A lightly boiled egg, cooked but still soft, is easily digested and suitable for the sick and for infants. The egg in its shell is placed gently into a pan of boiling water and kept boiling for three to four minutes.
- *Poached egg*: This too is suitable for those on a light diet. Break the shell, taking care not to break the egg-yolk, and pour the egg into the shallow pan of boiling water. Cook gently until the white part is opaque. Take it out with a flat spoon. It is usually served on a slice of toast with or without butter, and a little salt.
- *Albumen water*: The white of egg is only used. Separate the white from the yolk. Cut with a knife to break up the membrane and then add it to about 150 ml of water, stirring well or it may be mixed by shaking gently in a screw-topped jar. Strain before

serving, and add a little limejuice or glucose if desired.

- *Whey*: This is prepared from curds. It contains fats, sugars, salts and vitamins but no protein. Break up the curds with a fork and then drain off the whey by straining through gauze.

Feeding the Sick

The aim of feeding patients is to provide adequate nourishment to help and not to hinder restoration of health. In some cases artificial feeding (Feeding given other than through the mouth) may be necessary. Here we will deal with feeding the patients who are allowed to have food or fluids by mouth. An important responsibility of the nurse who is caring for the sick is to see that patients get the right diet at the proper time, to see that they take the food and to give necessary help in feeding helpless patients.

POINTS TO REMEMBER

- Meals for special diets must be served regularly and on time, making sure that the patient gets enough in 24 hours. Foods should be served hot as hot and cold as cold.
- Whenever possible, let patients have the foods they like best, but it should also be nutritious and suitable for their digestion.
- Prepare the environment. The ward should be quiet, well ventilated and free from all unpleasant sights and smells.
- Prepare the patient both mentally and physically to enjoy the food served. See that dressings or painful treatments are finished at least an hour before food is served.

  Help the patient to feel fresh and ready for the meal by washing face, hands and mouth. 5. Cleanliness of the food served and of all equipments is very important. The person serving the food must wear clean cloths and should have washed their hands well. Otherwise besides being distasteful to the patient, there is danger of introducing infection.

PROCEDURE - FEEDING THE PATIENT

- Prepare a covered tray containing the diet, drinking water, kidney tray, spoon, towel and a rubber sheet if needed.
- Help the patient into a comfortable position and arrange the towel to protect the clothing and bed linen.
- Talk with the patient, telling him what is being served.
- Make sure liquids are not too hot and use a feeding cup if needed. Ask the patient to open the mouth and pour it little.
- To give solids or soft diet, use a spoon and feed slowly, allowing the patient time to breathe and to masticate.
- When finished, give the patient some water to drink and to wash the mouth, receiving into the kidney tray.
- Wipe the lips with the towel, and leave the patient comfortable.
  Remove the tray, clean, dry and replace the articles.
- Record the time and amount of diet taken by the patient.

Procedure - Feeding the Children

- Children may eat best when allowed to sit at a small table with other children. Attractive coloured dishes and tumblers may help.
- Before the food is served, the hands and faces should be washed, and bibs tied on to protect clothing.
- It is the best if the mother helps her small child to feed.
- Serve little quantity at first and let the child have more if he will eat it.
- Encourage the child to finish the diet, but never force

a child to eat. Food should never be offered when a child is upset.

- Record the diet and time of food taken when the child has taken.
- Teach the child good eating habits when appropriate.

Ryle' s Tube-Feeding. (Refer Practicals) Purpose

To introduce liquid food through the nostril into the stomach, when the patient cannot or will not take food in the ordinary way. Some conditions are:

- When the patient is unconscious.
- Patients who are refusing food, e.g, in hysteria and mental illness.
- When the pharynx is paralyzed for any cause.
- After surgery of the mouth. 5. In Tetanus when there is difficulty in opening the mouth. 6. Premature babies who are too weak to suck.

Articles Required

- A sterile Ryle' s tube or naso-gastric tube.
- A 20 ml syringe.
- Lubricant such as liquid paraffin
- Litmus paper.
- Container of sterile water.
- Swab sticks
- Kidney tray
- Adhesive plaster
- Clip or spigot to close the end of the tube.
- Rubber or plastic sheet and treatment towel.
- Mouth wash if the patient can use it. Required feed in a measuring glass, a bowl of warm water (any liquid food that is strained and will pass through the tube with out blocking can be given).

Method

- Explain to the patient and get his co-operation.
- Position the patient usually sitting upright and supported.

- Bring the tray to the bedside and screen the bed.'
- Drape the plastic sheet and towel around the patient' s neck.
- Clear the nostril.
- Wash the hands then take the tube, lubricate it and make sure it is empty.
- Insert the tube along the floor of the nostril and gently pass it into the naso-pharynx.
- Ask the patient to swallow repeatedly while the nurse advance the tube quickly into the stomach.
- Attach the syringe to the end of the tube and aspirate the stomach contents.
- If there is doubt about the position of the tube, test the fluid aspirated with litmus paper. Blue litmus paper turns red when the tube is in the stomach, because of the acid in the gastric juice.
- Secure the tube to the nose or forehead with adhesive tape.
- If the patient can understand, talk to him about the food to be given as this may help his appetite and digestion.
- Before and after the feed introduce a little water. Ordered medicines may also be given through the tube.
- Give the food slowly. Instead of forcing it in through the syringe, the plunger may be removed and the food poured into the barrel.
- Give a mouthwash and make the patient comfortable with the tube clamped.
- Record the time, quantity and type of food given and the route.

Milk drip

If a milk drip is ordered, for eg. a patient with peptic ulcer, connect the nasogastric tube to a container of milk (covered) hung on a stand and use a drip bulb and clip to regulate the flow. See that the milk is fresh.

Index

O

P

Q

R

S

T

U

V

W

Z